REBOUND

Soaring in the NBA,
Battling Parkinson's,
and Finding What
Really Matters

Brian Grant and Ric Bucher

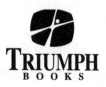

TRIUMPH
B O O K S

Library of Congress Cataloguing in Publication Data available upon request.

This book is available in quantity at special discounts for your group or organization. For further information, contact:

Triumph Books LLC
814 North Franklin Street
Chicago, Illinois 60610
(312) 337-0747
www.triumphbooks.com

Printed in U.S.A.
ISBN: 978-1-62937-811-4
Design by Patricia Frey

To the memory of: Kobe and Gianna Bryant—thank you, Kobe, for showing me what greatness is; Philippe Manicom, the best doctor I ever had; Mr. Martt, without whom no one would've ever heard of me; and Thomas E. Grant, my father, my friend, my hero.

—B.G.

To Brian Grant, for trusting me with his story and proving a big heart can overcome anything; my parents, Mathias and Helga Bucher, for showing me hard work and family devotion can achieve anything; to Corrine, Chance, and Mat, whose love means everything.

—R.B.

Contents

Foreword

I first ran in to Brian Grant in 1994 in Sacramento, California, where my mother lives to this day. I had just come home after finishing my last tour with Tony Toni Tone and BG had just been drafted by the Kings. I was a big fan of the team—the late Wayman Tisdale, a musician as well as a power forward, and I were good friends—but I knew a lot of NBA players weren't wild about being in Sacramento. When the Golden State Warriors traded Mitch Richmond to the Kings for Billy Owens back in 1991, I remember how unhappy Mitch looked. So when I ran in to Brian at a local sports bar, I was surprised when he immediately went into professional NBA-talk mode and said, "Nice to meet you, my brother, I'm thrilled to be a part of the community of Sacramento. My family and brother are all so excited about the Kings."

I was looking at him and wondering, *Why the ESPN answer?*
"Hey, man," I said, "I'm not that kind of fan."
He laughed. "Cool," he said.

Later that summer, I was riding my Harley Davidson down J Street, a pretty popular street in Sac. I pulled up next to BG sitting in a black Mercedes two-seater. The car was tough but too small for the big fella. BG asked me to join him at this Mexican restaurant, where the shots of tequila came fast and frequent. A few hours later, we were walking down the street and his then-girlfriend Gina called asking who the girl was that had left a message on his phone. He apparently had given Gina the code to retrieve his messages.

"Babe," he said. "You know who Raphael Saadiq is? Well, he's with me and his phone died so he gave the girl my number."

"Wait, what?" I said. I wish I could've seen the look on my face.

I found out later he did things like that just to get Gina to react. Her jealousy proved to him how much she loved him. We were boys from that day forward.

A lot of musicians and athletes connect, being performers and all, and I've been a hoops fan on the down-low for a long time. I wore a Mitch Richmond jersey in my "Ask of You" video and I got to know John "Spider" Salley in his Bad Boy days with the Pistons, but then Spider is cool with a lot of people. (Although I'm guessing he hasn't pulled a lot of other people onto the court during warm-ups to meet Michael Jordan, which he did for me.)

My relationship with BG, though, was different. I bought Kings courtside season tickets, but our connection went way beyond basketball.

Brian and I shared the same taste in music (everything from bossa nova to hip hop, and artists like Earth, Wind & Fire, Sade, and Neil Young). Ohio, where Brian is from, is a mecca for some of my favorite musicians and artists. He has a very good ear and hogs the playlist; to this day it's hard to get a song played in his house. I'm supposed to be the music aficionado, but he actually turned me on to listening to Pink Floyd's *Dark Side of the Moon* backwards. That's like me turning him on to Kareem Abdul-Jabbar's sky hook shot; it's not supposed to happen, but it did.

Brian's love for people is stronger than his love of music or basketball. I've watched him share his Parkinson's diagnosis with people from around the globe and it never fails to move me when I see the programs and fundraisers his foundation has created. The city of Portland, Oregon, has showed up for the man when he needed them most. I was so inspired I launched my own foundation, Recording Artists Advocating for Fairness (RAAF), to help artists with streaming rights.

I saw him connect with people who were struggling even before his diagnosis. I lived near the Kings' summer-run gym and one day passed Brian standing on the side of the road. A homeless man lying on the ground wrapped in blankets reading a book had piqued his curiosity, so he'd pulled his truck over to talk to him. Brian never carried the big-shot attitude with anyone and he didn't like to take advantage of his celebrity; I felt the same way. We'd go to these hot music clubs in San Francisco where the doormen would've let us right in, but unless it was cold or rainy, we were good with standing in line like everybody else.

Brian married Gina and the two of them did me the honor of naming me godfather of their second son, Jaydon "Boogie" Grant. I'm known as Uncle Ray to all eight of his kids and they've given me some of the funniest moments in my life.

Being part of the Grant family led to a visit to his hometown, Georgetown, which I learned is nothing like where I grew up in Oakland, California. Brian and I were in Georgetown, digging into a box of chili dogs at a famous local joint called Gold Star Chili, when an older White fella named Rex said, "Scoot over, boy," sat down next to me, and shoved me over with his butt.

I looked at Brian. I could tell he wasn't happy; I could also tell this wasn't the first time something like this had happened in Georgetown. We both let it go. After Rex left, Brian told me the man had purchased lettermen jackets for Brian's entire high school team his senior year; so I guess there's some good in everybody. But I'd never experienced anything like that in Oakland, that's for sure. It gave me a real introduction to what life must've been like for Brian growing up.

Fame and money were new for both of us. I had already learned some pretty hard lessons about handling the business end of my music career when we met and I wanted to save him from making the same mistakes—like setting up a living trust and not giving someone the power to write checks for you. I've been in the business 30-plus years and I still sleep with both eyes open, if you know what I mean. I took it as a compliment that his agent, Mark Bartelstein, wanted to meet me because he appreciated the advice I'd given Brian. Truth is, both Brian and I have had our share of struggles. The one constant is that we've been there for each other. That's what real ones do.

That, more than anything, defines who Brian is: A Real One. I'm glad that he decided to share his story, so you can find that out for yourself.

—*Grammy-winning recording artist Raphael Saadiq*

Introduction

My affinity for Brian Grant began long before he entrusted me to help him tell the world he was afflicted with young onset Parkinson's disease. Years before we ever met, I discovered we made it to the NBA in our respective fields having been born and raised in roughly the same part of southern Ohio. It's not exactly a well-worn path.

That two born-and-bred Buckeyes would collaborate to write a book as raw and deeply personal as this one also feels like quite an unlikely circumstance. If Midwesterners are known for anything, it's "holding our mud," as we like to say.

That said, there are a few characteristics that Brian and I share that might warrant our Midwesterner cards being revoked. Not the least of which is we both moved away.

The seed for this book was planted roughly 12 years ago, when I flew up from my home on the California coast and interviewed him at his palatial estate on the banks of the Willamette River just outside Portland, Oregon, his adopted home. With ESPN cameras and TV lights surrounding us, I thought about how far we both had come to cross paths in that moment.

I'm not talking just geographically but culturally as well.

When asked where I'm from and what it's like, I often joke that the tri-state area—southern Ohio, eastern Indiana, northern Kentucky—is a great place to grow up and settle down, but that it should be a law that everyone has to live somewhere else for at least a few years in between; largely, because it seems no one does. That I left to attend college in New Hampshire, got my first full-time job in San Diego, and have crisscrossed the country several times since makes me feel a bit like an oddball whenever I visit my hometown. Where most people from that part of the country might see it as a home base, from my early teens I saw it as a launching pad. When I go back, I'm sometimes asked about my life "out there," as if I've been on a mission into outer space. I viewed Brian as a fellow astronaut—and an oddball for another big reason.

Admitting personal flaws or weaknesses was not something I remember anyone ever doing during my time in southern Ohio. Too touchy-feely. Too vulnerable. I know from my conversations with Brian that he has a particularly strong aversion to conceding any sort of physical or mental weakness. Not only was he a mud-holding Midwestern boy, but he had spent more than a decade in the NBA at a time when it was far less progressive than it is today. No player then would have dreamed of admitting they suffered from depression, for example, as current NBA stars Kevin Love and DeMar DeRozan have in recent years. They would have feared being called "soft" and giving opponents a psychological advantage. The unwritten player code included topics you simply did not discuss—injuries, locker-room drama, drug use, and certainly not personal impropriety. No one was more dedicated to keeping all that in-house than Brian when he was playing.

Even if that house was bursting at the seams.

That's what struck me about Brian telling everyone he had Parkinson's—it wasn't something he *wanted* to do. He was clearly nervous as the cameras rolled, the jiggle of his arm becoming so pronounced that he grabbed his left wrist with his right hand to control it. When we were done, his shirt had half circles of sweat under his arms and a stripe down the back.

He resolutely set aside his fear of how the announcement might make people see him to offer something to those dealing with Parkinson's—the afflicted, family members, and caregivers alike. If there is a prevailing spirit about Brian, that might just be it. Other than to check facts, I wanted this book to be Brian's voice telling Brian's story, so I didn't quote any of the dozen or so other people I interviewed for it. But know this: every single former coach and teammate, unsolicited, talked about what a special teammate he was, how he dedicated himself to bucking them up off the court when they were struggling and supporting them with selfless play when they were on it. The NBA is a cutthroat, ego-driven place. In the 30 years I've covered it, I've come across a few relationships all the more special because they were forged in the fires of competition and I can't think of anyone more universally beloved and respected *as a person* than Brian.

That may be because of another Midwestern trait Brian has: he only wants what he has earned. Especially when it comes to respect. That is the essence of his reason for doing this book. If you are going to support his Parkinson's foundation, thank him for his contributions to your favorite team, praise his work with terminally ill kids, or express admiration for him in any way, it is important to him that you know exactly who he is in full. In typical Brian fashion, he didn't go halfway on that once he committed to it, either. He was adamant about not exposing anyone else's skeletons in this book, but he bravely pulled his out of the closet and revealed every bone and crevice.

That, of course, included the circumstances that led to Brian fathering children with four different women. It screams of the stereotypical careless, self-indulgent professional athlete and that's not who I know Brian to be.

One of the first times we sat down to discuss this book, he told me that Parkinson's disease and the side effects of some of the medications left him with memory issues, both short- and long-term. He could walk into a shop, walk back out, and have no idea where he parked his car. I also knew that his bouts of depression—another symptom—made him difficult to reach, sometimes for weeks at a time.

On one of Brian's visits—pre-pandemic—to work on the book, he shared with me an incident in the lobby of his hotel, where he had gone to grab a cup of coffee from a self-serve station. He noticed a woman staring at him with a look of pity as he battled his jiggling arm to prepare his cup without making a mess. "Parkinson's," he said to the lady, smiling.

"Oh, no," she said. "I…."

I could empathize with both the lady's discomfort and Brian's in having to smile in the face of strangers pitying him, when, not that long ago, they gazed at him in awe. To see the same man I had watched fearlessly stare down countless opponents on the court look so vulnerable was unnerving. Losing control of some part of ourselves, I believe—be it an arm, bladder, or mental faculties—is a universal fear that only grows as we get older. To see someone exhibiting that very thing inspires the reflexive thought: *What's wrong with them?* Followed by, *That's so sad.*

As I've learned from Brian, that reaction might be understandable but it's nevertheless demoralizing. Answer to the first question: Nothing, other than their brain has stopped producing the normal amount of dopamine. Response to the second remark: No, that's life.

I understood that thanks to my other kinship with Brian.

I, too, have waged my own battle with addiction. I've felt the shame of allowing a substance to subvert my best intentions and make me behave in ways that hurt family and friends. I've learned how to keep those demons at bay successfully for more than 30 years now, but I've never forgotten that first time, at someone's suggestion, I looked into my own eyes in a mirror and saw how much sadness and regret they held.

Despite all that, I wasn't quite sure I wanted to write this book. Or, rather, that this book needed to be written. Writing a book is a hard, arduous endeavor; I didn't want to put myself or Brian through what it would take unless I knew it would serve a greater purpose.

The prevalence of Parkinson's, and what Brian is looking to do for his fellow sufferers, offered that. Within the last two years, my father-in-law was diagnosed with it and legendary Utah Jazz coach Jerry Sloan reportedly died from it. I know former Orlando Magic GM John Gabriel, who is living with it. I was repeatedly surprised by people I told about this project who knew or were related to someone with Parkinson's. Overall, 10 million people in the world have it, and 60,000 more are diagnosed every year in the U.S. alone.

Of all the insights and revelations Brian shared with me, there's one that is threaded through all of them—from the drive to get away from the Ohio river bank, to his against-all-odds road to the NBA, his drama-filled 12-year career, his dive into Rastafarianism, his drug addiction, his acceptance of his Parkinson's and his search for purpose after:

Gina. He's never forgiven himself for finding, and then losing "the love of his life," his first wife and mother to four of his children.

His behavior and the consequences cut him so deeply that he says he never has been unfaithful in any of his subsequent relationships. I believe him, in part because he is so honest and forthcoming about all his other shortcomings, including a few he still hasn't conquered.

That, for me, is what makes this book truly redemptive. It's not just a catalogue of Brian's many gut-torquing ups and downs and how he survived them, but how they've revealed who he is at heart. It has been said that wealth doesn't change people, it just makes them more of who they always were. I would say the same applies to hardships; success doesn't reveal our true nature, challenges do.

My perception of bravery and resilience and devotion to family have been reshaped by having helped Brian tell his story. I hope reading it does the same for you.

—Ric Bucher
December 2020

REBOUND

chapter 1
Tremors and Volcanoes

I had to ask.

What I hoped to hear: "It's nothing." Or, at least: "It's nothing to worry about." That's what I hoped.

Deep down, though, I had a feeling I wasn't going to get the answer I wanted. If that sounds pessimistic, well, there was a reason: at that moment, nothing in my life was going the way I wanted.

From the outside, it might not have seemed that way. Newly retired from a rewarding 12-year career in the NBA, I had all the perks that come with it, both materially and personally. Big houses in Portland and Miami and a getaway cabin in the woods of Oregon. A fishing boat. A bank account fat enough that, if I was smart, I'd never have to work again. A beautiful wife, Gina, my one true love, a great mother to our four kids and a former dancer who still looked very much like a dancer, if you know what I mean.

I had worked my ass off for two of the most loyal franchises in the league—the Portland Trail Blazers and Miami Heat—that assured I'd be welcome even though I no longer grabbed rebounds for them. Even though I wasn't playing anymore, I was recognized wherever I went—I guess that's to be expected when you're a 6'9" Black man who is the spitting image of Rasta legend Bob Marley. I even had an American bulldog, Brutus, that liked to chew up my shoes and drown me in sloppy wet kisses. For a Black kid from a little farming town on the banks of the Ohio River who expected to be in a field picking tobacco and potatoes his whole life, that's a pretty amazing step-up.

Dig just a little ways below the surface, though, and things were a lot different. It wasn't just that the six-figure paychecks were no longer rolling in every two weeks. Or that I no longer had crowds cheering and chanting my name on a nightly basis. Or that I was no longer officially part of the NBA, flying around the country on private jets and staying in five-star hotels and having beautiful women handing me their phone number. Having all that go away is something every professional athlete has to deal with when they retire.

It felt as if I was dealing with something heavier. I had ridden an elevator in the building of life to a floor way higher than I ever thought possible for someone like me. At the moment, though, I was out on the ledge of that high-rise, hanging on by my fingers—and starting to lose my grip.

The marriage to that beautiful woman? I'd fucked that up. The standing welcome I had from my former teams? I went to a game and sat in the stands and the people around me were so polite. "Congratulations, man, and thank you for the work you put in here," one fan said. But by halftime I was so anxious my heart was pounding and I was squirming in my seat. My head and my body were telling me, "You're supposed to be out there working right now because this is when we work." I didn't realize I would miss it as much as I did. I left and never went back.

The willpower that allowed me to beat the odds, make it to the NBA, and out-work bigger, stronger men also seemed to have disappeared. It felt like there was a black cloud hanging over me and some monstrous weight sitting on my shoulders from the minute I opened my eyes every morning—a psychological weight that was turning into very real pounds around my waist. I love to fish and now I had all the time in the world to do it. Friends invited me to go out on their boats all the time, but they and Gina would practically have to drag me to the docks. I eventually stopped leaving the house, preferring to sit on my couch in the dark watching people fish on my TV screen while I felt sorry for myself and self-medicated with the opioids I had left over from the multitude of surgeries during my playing days.

Those who knew me from my playing days would've never imagined me living like that. Hell, I never imagined it, either.

Throughout my playing career, Gina had done everything possible to make life easier. She understood the competitive world in which I lived, the razor-thin difference between having a job in the NBA and all the perks that came with it and being just another tall Black man in search of a job.

Now it was my turn to make life easier for her. She was starting her career as a fitness dance instructor, something that made her feel good about herself, something that she could claim as her own beyond being the mother of our children and supporting me and my career. Did I support her the way she supported me? No. I was jealous and paranoid. Day after day I'd sit on the couch, eat bowls of Cap'n Crunch Berries, watch TV, and call her every bad name in the book. I accused her of being unfaithful and of caring more about her career than me. I was never physical with her but I'm sure I frightened her; a man as big as me on a rampage, throwing dishes and smashing pictures will do the trick. I had learned how to channel my rage and pain to attack the basket and intimidate men bigger and stronger than me. I even had thousands cheering me for it. But that was in the middle of a big arena. Acting like that in the confines of our home was a lot different.

Truth is, Gina wanted to figure out what the hell was going on with me and how she could help. She tried to get me out of the house or have friends over. But I was stuck between being consumed with guilt over how I was acting and outraged over what I thought she was doing behind my back.

The last thing I wanted was to drive Gina away; the fear that I might lose her fueled my anger. I suspected I was dealing with something more than post-retirement funk, but I didn't want anyone to know, least of all her. I had always considered myself the family rock, the strong one, the one who overcame whatever stood in front of me to take care of my family. She did, too, leaving notes in my shaving kit to find on road trips that said exactly that: "Thank you for taking care of our family, my shining star." So it was on me to figure this out. I didn't want to hear anything about depression. That was for the weak, or the weak-minded, and I had proved over and over again I was anything but that.

It took six months for me to admit to Gina that I was depressed and then another three months before I made a doctor's appointment to do something about it. Pride can be a pretty tough opponent. Sensing that Gina was ready to give up on me and our marriage finally got me to seek medical help; her threatening to leave and take the kids with her if I didn't see a doctor might've given me that sense. I never imagined being someone in a psychiatrist's office, talking about feeling lost and bawling my eyes out, but there I was. The psychiatrist also prescribed me an anti-depressant, Zoloft, which helped me start to reconnect with my friends and actually leave the house.

Adding the Zoloft helped balance my body's chemistry, but there was still something going on that I wasn't aware of—dopamine.

Philippe Manicom was one of the first people I let back into the house. To call him merely a massage therapist or acupuncturist wouldn't do him justice, but those were the talents that made him a popular figure within a circle of world-famous celebrities based in Miami—Julio Iglesias, Marc Anthony, Lenny Kravitz, and my old enemy Shaquille O'Neal, to name-drop a few. So, when it came time to stop ignoring a physical tic that had grown progressively stronger during my self-imposed hibernation, Philippe seemed like the natural person to ask. We were sitting next to each other on a plane, flying back from Portland to Miami, when I rolled my arm over and pointed to a tiny patch of twitching skin near my left wrist.

"Hey, Philippe," I said, "what do you think this is?"

I had asked the question once before, almost a year earlier, but not to him. I was still in the NBA at the time, winding down my career with the Phoenix Suns, when I pointed it out to the team athletic trainer.

"B, you're just getting old, man, but we can go see the neurologist and have him check it out," he said. The team neurologist had a similar diagnosis—a muscle twitching from years of over-use. "I suspect you're going to see a lot of that in different places, because you've been in the league so long," he said. "You've had a good run and you played hard and been beat up." And with that, I didn't think anything more about it.

Every year there are 60 players—selected out of hundreds of thousands—added to the mix through the NBA draft. Those of us already in the league will take anything, do anything, try anything, to keep our spot. Playing through pain becomes necessary, or at least it was for me; I needed 14 major surgeries to get through my 12 years. I had learned to negotiate with my body: *Just get me through this and we'll fix whatever needs to be fixed in the off-season.* I wasn't alone. Everyone—coaches, GMs, athletic trainers, owners—learns to see players as somehow above the laws of normal human beings. Because in a lot of ways, NBA players are. Guys our size aren't supposed to be as fast or jump as high or have the endurance we have. It might not be apparent when you're watching on your TV screen or even when you're in the stands, because everyone on the court is unusually big and fast. But put one average-sized human with average athleticism out there and the difference would be obvious—shoot, the difference when an NBA player declines just a little bit is pretty apparent.

Because it takes a combination of size, athleticism, and mental toughness that is rare, an NBA team will provide every resource imaginable to keep someone with all those traits functioning. Some physical quirk that might be a red flag for the average Joe is often viewed as just the price of business for a player in the NBA.

But what had been a damn twitch on my wrist in Phoenix now occasionally included a wiggly pinkie finger. As much as I wanted to still believe this was merely a side effect from the physical grind of 12 NBA seasons, I thought, *Shouldn't it be getting better, not worse?* It had been a year since my body had last endured an NBA game or practice. I knew plenty of professional athletes, including a few former teammates, say how much better their bodies felt once they stopped playing; that wasn't happening for me, mentally or physically. If anything, I felt worse. It felt like my entire life was sliding in the wrong direction. I was losing control—over my marriage, my weight, and even my general outlook on life. All of it symbolized by a pinkie finger suddenly with a mind of its own.

I had come to respect Philippe, both for his knowledge of what makes bodies work the way they do—especially mine—as well as his honesty. I considered him a friend. I hoped he was going to tell me the skin tremor was related to some issue of flexibility or diet or nerve endings, something we had discussed or he had treated me for in the past. Something fixable.

He turned and looked at me as if he'd been waiting a long time for me to ask.

"Brian," he said, "I love you too much not to tell you."

I studied his face. "What is it?"

"I'm going to tell you what you have."

"What I have? What do I have?"

"You have Parkinson's."

"What? Don't say no shit like that!"

Parkinson's? It was as if Philippe had punched me in the face.

I wasn't even sure exactly what Parkinson's was; all I knew was that it was really bad and that Michael J. Fox had it, and the only reason I knew that was because I was a big fan of his, going all the way back to his first TV sitcom, *Family Ties*. For a disease to take over the system of a short, slightly-built actor, okay—but someone built like me, in his thirties, who could dunk on the heads of 7-footers? There was no way I could be afflicted with the same disease as Marty McFly.

"Brian, let me see your hands," Philippe said calmly. First he flexed my left hand back at the wrist and then released it; it shuddered, as if it were being cranked back into place. Then he did the same with my right hand, and when he did, my hand naturally flopped forward.

"You see that?" he said. "That's the beginning of it. And you were depressed for nine months, right? Usually that comes before everything else."

He could tell I was still looking for a reason not to believe him.

"Let me do it again," he said. He pushed the fingers of my left hand back toward my shoulder and let go; same shudder. "You see how that is?" To eliminate any thought I might have that the difference might be my right hand being my dominant one, he demonstrated on his two hands. When he released them, they both flopped forward. "This is how they should look," he said.

Pride in my strength and endurance went back to my days picking crops and it only grew with each monstrous dunk or rebound or 300-pound center I stopped in his tracks. I was a gifted athlete, but I wasn't a freak by NBA standards; it was my will, or my motor, as basketball scouts like to say, that served as my secret weapon. I could've been a small forward but in my relatively short pre-NBA career—one year in high school, four in college—I'd always been a big man playing around the basket. The only basketball camp I ever attended was a free week-long one at my high school essentially available to whoever signed up. No AAU tournaments or shoe-sponsored skills camps or hoop summits for me. My skills were decent for a big man, but I'd never developed the ball-handling and long-range shooting skills needed to play small forward. On the other hand, I was slightly undersized at that time for being a power forward. I had to work harder than most of my opponents to offset some natural advantage they had over me—speed, size, skill.

Along the way, I'd seen my body suffer all kinds of consequences yet eventually recover, proof you can get used to almost anything. That's what I learned: no setback is permanent, no injury is insurmountable. I took pride in that—my athleticism and my willingness to push my body to its limits had earned me a lot of money, attention, and admiration. It was my identity. No longer being able to showcase that in front of thousands of cheering fans undoubtedly was part of my funk. But this—this was well beyond that. Now I was being told that I was disabled, impaired, that my hand couldn't do something every hand should.

My self-worth had taken a few heavy hits over the last year. I wasn't the athlete I once was. I wasn't the husband or father I hoped to be. I hadn't been much of a friend lately. But this? This wasn't a bad attitude, it was a broken operating system. Philippe might as well have told me I was deformed.

"Man, you can't tell me that!" I barked, wild-eyed. "You don't know what I've got."

Philippe just looked at me and shook his head. "Brother, I've treated a lot of people," he said quietly. "I wouldn't lie to you because I love you. But don't worry—I have a plan. I'll make you better. I'm going to take you to Dominica. It's an island right next to Guadeloupe where I grew up. I'm going to take you there and we're going to heal you. We're going to clean your blood so that the Parkinson's doesn't progress. You can live a long time with this."

I was still in a daze from Philippe's diagnosis when I walked in my front door. It tells you a lot about the state of my marriage that I didn't say anything to Gina about Philippe's diagnosis. I had been so miserable she had no way of knowing that something brand new was weighing on my mind. When I finally did talk to her, I simply said, "I'm going to an island called Guadeloupe with Philippe to try to heal."

Keep in mind, I had just come out of a nine-month depression. During that whole time, she had singlehandedly raised our four kids—Jaydon, Elijah, Maliah, and Anaya—and built her career as a Zumba instructor, a fitness regime that was quickly becoming a global hit—all while trying to steer clear of her large, angry, moody husband.

I wasn't only depressed and envious that she was now the hot ticket, I was scared and suspicious. I knew all about the temptations of the road. Gina had found out in the first months of our relationship my capacity to be unfaithful, and in my twisted state of mind I convinced myself she was now going to get back at me. Right before Philippe and I left for the airport, I finally told her that Philippe thought I might have Parkinson's. Even that didn't stir much of a reaction. I couldn't blame her, in light of the previous nine months, but it still hurt. Maybe she didn't believe me and thought I was off on some boys' weekend. Or she was so worn down dealing with me that it just didn't matter. For now, it was good enough that I'd be out of the house. "Just go," she said.

I'd made the trip to Portland to check on the house I still had there, but it was a reminder of happier times and what Gina and I had left behind. We had never intended on making Miami our home. We loved being in Portland and I loved playing for the Blazers, but after being good enough to get to the Western Conference finals two years in a row but not good enough to get any further, I knew our GM, Bob Whitsitt, would try to do something with the roster to take that final step. He also had a potential free agent with a solid reputation whose contract could be shaped to make a trade—me.

That's how I wound up in Miami playing for the Heat and crossing paths with Philippe.

He pegged me for someone who needed some physical help the very first time we met. I was midway through my career but had already had major surgery on both knees and both shoulders. I don't want to sound cynical, but if you're a professional athlete, you get a lot of people offering their help and it's hard to know what the person's motive is. Sometimes they genuinely recognize you have a problem and want to help solve it. More often, though, they are looking for a way into the exclusive and lucrative world of professional sports. They know who you are, know you have a lot of money, and want to find a way to get some of it. I learned all that the hard way; not having received star treatment in high school or college, I wasn't used to people trying to exploit me. My natural inclination is to connect with people and trust them, but being burned a few times sent me the other direction—I became wary of everyone. Most of the time, when someone offered their help, a sarcastic voice in my head would say, "Suurrrre you can."

I had developed a routine in Miami of swinging by the marina in Coconut Grove, not far from my house, to buy fresh fish off the charter-boat captains who took tourists out on half-day fishing excursions. That's where this skinny White dude in aviator glasses, looking as if he'd just walked off the set of *Miami Vice*, walked up to me and said, "Brother, I've been trying to get a hold of you. Here's a flyer. I would love to put my hands on you."

For a second I thought he was propositioning me and I started to see red. "What the fuck are you talking about?" I said.

"No, man, not like that," he said, with an accent I'd learn later was French-Creole. "I'd like to do some healing. I do acupuncture and massage." The flyer was the kind you see taped up on telephone poles and bulletin boards. I'd actually seen a stack of them at the Heat facilities. Let's just say people with Phillipe's résumé and client list usually aren't handing out flyers.

He talked as if he knew me, which also made me wary. He told me I was very popular on the island where he was born, Guadeloupe, as well as on the surrounding islands. Sounds like a con job, right? I'd never heard of any of the islands, much less ever been to one of them. How could I possibly be popular there?

His pitch didn't get past my skepticism, especially when he said he did acupuncture as part of his treatment. That killed any chance he might have had. He might as well have said to me straight out, "I'm a scam artist." Because when I started my career in Sacramento I met an acupuncturist who put his needles in me, attached little electrodes to them, and said, "See? See how the muscles are jumping?"

"Yeah," I said. "That's muscle stimulation."

"No, no, those are the meridians." He wanted me to believe he was tapping into a Chinese medicine concept about the body having 12 meridians or channels of energy that flow through the body.

"Whatever, man," I said. "You're a quack." It pissed me off that he considered me that gullible. I thought, *Dude, I play on a professional team. I get this kind of treatment every day. You're not doing shit.* I didn't say that out loud. I just left when he was done, never went back, and swore off acupuncture as the work of snake oil salesmen.

So I took one of Philippe's flyers and promised to call him only to be nice. Of course, the next time I went to the marina, I ran in to him again. He, too, loved buying fresh fish off the boats. "You should call me, mon," he said. "I could really help you."

At that point, I needed help from someone. As anybody who has played for legendary coach Pat Riley will tell you, his conditioning demands are no joke. I was always known for my willingness to play hard and outwork my opponent on any given night, but Pat asked more of me than any other coach I ever had. I knew he would, which is why at first I had no interest in playing for him or the Heat. As a coach, he had a reputation for long, grueling practices. When championships were the result, as it was with the Lakers, players felt they were worth it. Even as the coach in New York, he took the Knicks to the NBA Finals. Riley's first six years in Miami, the Heat went to the playoffs every year, but they only made it out of the first round twice. That wasn't enough, in a lot of players' minds, to offset the extra years they thought Riley would grind off of them.

What they didn't know—as I didn't, at first—is that as much as Riley asked his players to give him, he was willing to give even more in return. He also knew firsthand that toughness and effort, every day, all day, could trump any other advantage. Most guys who averaged 7.4 points shooting barely over 40 percent would not last more than a season or two in the NBA; but those were Riley's career numbers and he lasted nine seasons. He even won a championship as a player with the Lakers, coming off the bench as a defensive fireplug and serving as a practice dummy for the team's star guard, Jerry West.

Which is why I gave him everything I had and never thought twice about what it might cost. A decision I never regretted, even though I was never quite the same after playing in Miami.

It might've been different if we played the game then the way it is played now, but the NBA has changed a lot in the last 20 years. The biggest shift is in the size of the players—small ball rules the league these days. LeBron James is my height, 6'9", and is often the tallest player on the court, sometimes by an inch or two. I *never* came close to being the biggest player on the floor.

Riley did not believe in small ball, at least not then, but he transformed me into a center, mostly out of necessity. His coaching philosophy seemed to be, "It's not the size of the dog in the fight, it's the size of the fight in the dog." Alonzo Mourning, at 6'10" and 260 pounds, was undersized for a center in those days but became an All-Star not only with an appetite for bruising physical contact and a perfectly chiseled physique, but a stare that could blister paint. I was supposed to play power forward next to him.

Thirteen games into the season, a kidney disease sidelined Zo and I became our big man—even though I was not big at all by NBA standards. Or my own. I had trimmed down to 248 pounds, a good 20 pounds below my normal playing weight, at the recommendation of the Heat's strength and conditioning coach, Bill Foran. Riley trusted Bill completely and allowed him to set weight and body mass index marks for every player. If you didn't meet them, you had to do extra conditioning until you did. Mine were 255 and 11 percent BMI. Some guys, if they were worried about making their marks when it came time for

Bill to use the calipers to measure their body fat, would offer a bribe: *C'mon, Bill, let me wash the car or something.*

It made sense to put less weight on my surgically repaired knees, but it put me at an extreme disadvantage at my new position. Centers at that time were almost all 7 feet or taller and weighed an *average* of 260 pounds. I was battling Shaq, Arvydas Sabonis (7'3", 279), Big Country Reeves (7', 275) and Erick Dampier (6'11", 265), to name a few. Not every center I faced was an All-Star, of course, but nearly every one of them was bigger and heavier and the NBA allowed players to throw their weight around then in a way they don't now. I tried to make up the difference by making them chase me around the court on offense, but on defense I still had to keep my body between them and the basket. The fight in this dog had to be huge, because the dog, relatively, was not.

Adding weight during the season wasn't something I could do, either; not good weight, as in muscle, anyway. The grind of the season is more likely to cause you to lose five to 10 pounds. Whether I gave the beating or took it—and there were centers like Ben Wallace (6'9", 240) and Jermaine O'Neal (6'11", 226) where it was more of a fair fight—every muscle and joint in my body paid the price. All of which left me thinking I should roll the dice and take up Philippe on his offer.

In movies, there's the sound of a church choir when the heavens open or something miraculous happens. That's what

I felt the first time Philippe worked on me. He started with a massage and every knotted muscle and screaming tendon disappeared. Usually when you're working with a new masseuse, it takes them a couple of sessions to get to know the parts of your body that need the most attention; sometimes you have to tell them. Not Philippe. As he worked on me that first time, he immediately identified where I was hurting the most and went from the connective tissue deep into the muscle.

"I want to break out my needles now," he said.

I tensed up again as soon as I heard the word "needles." I reminded him about my previous experience with acupuncture; he asked me to give him a chance. The massage had been so good, how could I argue?

I was lying on my back when he put one needle in my ear and another between my eyebrows. Then he started to twist the second one. I thought the massage had relaxed my body but that twisting needle took me to a whole other level. It happened so fast that I'm sure someone watching would've thought it was fake; but the truth is, he literally put me to sleep.

Giving Philippe a chance to work on me was one of the best decisions I've ever made. I got so much more than just relief from my aches and pains. I came to truly understand what Chinese medicine was all about through Philippe. He knew it all—acupuncture, the herbs, everything. I found out later he had been appointed the medical ambassador for Dominica, the island next to Guadeloupe. It also turned out he lived 15 minutes from me in Miami. Every time I had a heavy game or a particularly hard practice and I couldn't sleep because I was hurting so badly, I'd call him. He'd come over and set up his table. One needle in my ear, one between my eyebrows. One twist each and after he let go of the second one I was out—every time. The acupuncture became routine, along with a massage and moxibustion—using burning herbs to heat the skin near an injured area. I didn't understand the science behind everything he was doing but he clearly did. He was the real deal.

There was only one problem: I wasn't the only one who knew he was gifted. All the top entertainers in Miami knew who Philippe was and highly respected his magic healing touch as well. That included Shaquille O'Neal—although it's hard to imagine anybody he played made him ache as much as he did them. Philippe didn't just work on athletes, either. Big-time, Miami-based musical artists Timbaland and Marc Anthony swore by him. Mama B, the mother of Bob Marley, considered him her primary physician. Just about every Miami-based star you can think of had Philippe on speed dial.

I didn't know just how popular he was when we first met because if you were getting treated by him you didn't want to help add to his list of clients; that would only make it harder to see him. I went from someone who thought acupuncture was a hoax to trying to convince Philippe to go see Timbaland *after* he stuck his needles in me.

Philippe was also a good soul; it felt good just to be around him. And if there's one thing that should become crystal clear for anyone reading this, I can become obsessed with things that make me feel good. When I retired, quite a few things were no longer available to me and fell off that list. I wasn't about to let Philippe become one of them.

When I agreed to go to Dominica, I did it without really knowing where I was going or how we were getting there. That last part proved to be an adventure in itself. We flew a regular commercial jet from Miami to San Juan, Puerto Rico, and then took a small 12-seat prop plane from there to the island. Life in the islands might be laid back, but getting there definitely is not. As you approach the island, it looks as if you're going to fly into a mountain. Once you clear that, the plane drops straight down until its skimming above banana trees. A very short runway suddenly appears, the plane touches down, and the pilot slams on the brakes to keep from skidding into the ocean. I took off for Dominica hoping it would cure me of a deadly disease. Before I got off the plane, I wondered if it might kill me instead.

Once we touched down, I found out that Philippe was even more popular in the islands than he was in Miami. Everyone knew him. I also went from considering him a friend and a naturopath, but not a real doctor—which meant there was a chance, in my mind, that his diagnosis was off—to something more. I quickly learned he was essentially the minister of health for the three islands. Everybody greeted him as "Dr. Manicom." I also found out that he had not been lying about my popularity, either. Bobby, the island's director of tourism and a Bob Marley look-alike, met us at the airport and said, "The Local Dreads, they love you. You're a superstar here."

It wasn't just the dreads. When we stopped at a little shack on the side of the road to buy a soda, there was a group of kids playing basketball across the street on a makeshift court with a milk crate for a basket.

As I stepped out of the car, one of the kids said, "Hey, Brian Grant, you want to get a game?"

I'm in the middle of nowhere, somewhere I've never been before, in regular clothes, and the kid instantly recognized me. I'm not sure what I appreciated more: the invitation, or the confidence that they thought they could hang with a former NBA player. "No, but thank you," I said. "Y'all would beat me."

It was the same everywhere I went—the people inside the store greeted me by name, as did the fans at a local soccer match we stopped to watch. They truly thought I was one of their own. "Brian, what island are you from?" they asked. I told them I grew up near the water, but I wasn't from any island. It wasn't just my dreads and goatee that made them think I was one of them, either. They had seen me play on TV and identified with my quiet but physical style.

"You don't just look like you're from the islands, mon," they said in their sing-song tropical lilt. "You play like it, too."

One of the biggest attractions on Dominica is a natural hot spring called Boiling Lake, which I'm told is the second-largest hot spring in the world. Like a lot of tourist attractions, it proved to sound way more impressive than it looked. It was more of a volcanic puddle than a lake. We didn't soak in it; the nearby villa we stayed in piped water from it into a little lagoon on the property. If that sounds fancy, trust me, it wasn't. When they wanted to fill the lagoon, they simply opened a faucet and hot "lake" water came shooting out of a pipe. It was not a high-tech operation.

"What prevents scalding hot water from coming out of that pipe?" I asked.

"Nothing," Philippe said, grinning.

We had just started soaking in the lagoon when a kid came up to Philippe and looked at him expectantly. This clearly was not the first time he'd been here. "What color mud you need?" he asked.

He described several different types of mud and handed the kid $20. He disappeared into the jungle and returned about 20 minutes later with plastic bags of yellow, brown, and red mud. Philippe explained to me how each mud contained a different kind of mineral and what each could do for me by having them absorbed through my skin.

"We're going to put this all over you," he said.

As much as I wanted to believe that what Philippe was doing would help me, I felt self-conscious sitting there having him rub mud all over me. It didn't help that two other local couples were soaking in the lagoon with us, watching intently. Or that Philippe and I were both in our underwear as he talked to me in a low voice and slathered me with mud.

"Hurry up," I said.

He must've thought I was in a rush to feel the effects of the mud.

"Be patient," he said.

"Hurry up," I repeated. I was obviously used to having Philippe's hands on me, but for whatever reason—the sun, the hot water, the goopy mud—this felt more sensual. I'd never had him work on me outside with someone watching, either. The people watching us weren't sure what to make of the mud bath, either; clearly they hadn't seen this ritual before. At one point, one of the people watching us asked, "You guys alright? Is that mud he's rubbing on you?"

"Yeah, brother," Philippe said. "We're good."

"This is healing mud. *Healing* mud," I emphasized.

I got the sense that Philippe knew he was making me uncomfortable—and was getting a kick out of it. He finally looked over at the couples watching and then at me and understood. "Oh, mon, don't worry about that," he said. "You like the women. I like the women. Forget them."

How did it feel? Pretty much the way you'd expect warm mud to feel. When we were finally done, we walked over to a natural waterfall and rinsed off in the cold, clear water.

Did it help? I want to say it did, but it was hard to separate the effects of the mud from the general therapeutic value of being on a tropical island. The warm air, the easygoing lifestyle, the fresh air and food and the friendliness of the people made me forget about all that I missed about the NBA. I came to believe the volcano's healing powers had as much to do with the environment as anything else. We were essentially living in a jungle where someone had taken a machete and carved a few streets out of it. Everything we ate was grown or raised on the island. The air and water were clean. We visited a little village where there were multiple women who were 113 years old or older. The oldest was 121. Philippe spoke Creole, French, and English and asked one of them in Creole the secret to her old age. They spoke for a minute and then he translated. "She says she never eats anything that isn't from the island," he said. "If she eats meat, it was raised on the island. If she eats vegetables, they were grown on the island."

Everyone, young and old, was relaxed. I usually listen to music as an escape, a way to chill, but down there I didn't need it. I'd fall asleep to the sounds of the wildlife in the bushes and trees just outside my window.

I'd never seen a night sky filled with so many stars, either; it looked like something out of a movie. I slept better than I had in a long time and when I woke up, I wasn't lethargic the way I was at home. I stopped worrying about my failing marriage and how I was going to get better physically. The twitch in my finger practically disappeared.

I was so grateful for the way the island people treated me, I helped them fix their outdoor basketball court. It actually wasn't a court, anymore, but a pasture for goats, who fed on the weeds and grass that had sprouted up through the cracks in the asphalt. We did it up right. I had backboards and goals shipped over from Miami. We bulldozed the old asphalt, laid down a fresh surface, and painted the standard court lines on it. We even added three rows of bleachers and a little wooden shack as a press box.

After I got back to Miami from that first trip, my relaxed state and reduced tremor lasted for a few days. I was in such a better mood, Gina said, "Wow, you might need to go down there more often." About three weeks later I did go back and took her with me, where we discovered one of the few downsides to island life. Everything is open air—no AC, no screens—with lizards running across the floor. Those didn't bother me. But when we fell asleep we forgot to pull down the mosquito netting canopy above the bed. We woke up in the middle of the night covered in those suckers. Despite that—or maybe as a reflection of how bad things had become—it was one of the better times in the final days of our marriage.

Every time I got back to Miami, though, the island effect would last about three or four days and then I'd be right back in the same dark head space I had before I left. Bitter ol' Brian, my alter ego, would return and make everyone miserable. Including me. Part of me wondered if I should just move to the islands for good, but that would be giving up—on my marriage, on my kids, and on finding a passion and a purpose now that I didn't play basketball anymore. I wasn't ready to do any of that.

I still had hope that Philippe's diagnosis had been wrong and that there was another explanation for my tremor, so when we got back from that first island trip I made an appointment with the Heat's neurologist. When I walked in he could tell right away that something was wrong. I was not anything like the happy and confident Brian Grant he had last seen playing for the Heat. I was talking a million miles an hour about everything—how Gina and I weren't getting along, how I was gaining weight, how lost I felt not playing anymore. He attributed it all to depression. When I finally stopped talking, he prescribed Zoloft, an anti-depressant. "You could have Parkinson's, but your friend was wrong to tell you that," he said. "It could be something else. Let's see how the Zoloft works first. The tremor could just be stress."

Of course, I didn't tell him everything. He was giving me the answer I wanted and I wasn't about to try to convince him he was wrong. His diagnosis might've changed had I mentioned what happened my last year playing for the Suns.

Truth is, I didn't play a whole lot in Phoenix. Not in actual games, anyway. The coach, Mike D'Antoni, was known for having the team play at a very fast pace, in order to create as many offensive possessions and shots as possible. D'Antoni wanted to get up a shot in seven seconds or less every time we had it. I would've loved that style when I first got to the league; at 34, I was the second-oldest player on the team. After playing in nine of our first 13 games, I didn't play again until March. The most action I saw was in practice. NBA rules allow teams to have a maximum of 12 players available for a game, but coaches usually don't use more than eight on any given night. The four at the end of the bench try to stay ready by playing games of two-on-two or one-on-one after the regular team practice. I was now one of those guys, along with another veteran, Kurt Thomas. We were the old heads, keeping each other in shape. One day, late in the season, I blew by him for a layup, went to jump off my left leg to dunk it, and lost my balance. But it wasn't like just normal losing your balance; it was as if the strength in my leg suddenly disappeared. Not only had I never felt anything like it, I'd never seen anything like it. It was so odd everyone in the gym stopped and stared. Kurt scrunched up his face.

"What happened?" he asked.

I tried to play it off. "Yo, did I miss?"

"Miss? You looked like you were about to break your damn neck! You went up all crazy." That's when I realized I couldn't jump off my left leg as well as I once could.

It's humbling enough, as a pro athlete, to realize you can't move the way you once could. The simple things that came so naturally now took serious effort or concentration—or no longer could be done. Sometimes it happens all at once, but more often the decline is gradual, subtle. You go to sprint past a defender and find you can't. You jump to grab a ball and you're a second late or the ball grazes your fingertips, when previously you'd have snatched it with both hands. All that was happening to me, but this was not that. This was the equivalent of walking down the street and falling flat on your face.

I played it off at the time, chalking it up to the athletic trainer's theory that it was a by-product of running into and wrestling with men much bigger than me on a nightly basis for more than a decade. But I never forgot that it happened or how strange it felt. And it wasn't a one-time thing, it was just the only time it was so obvious others noticed.

I neglected to mention any of that to the Heat doctor. Then again, I wasn't in search of the truth; I was in search of an answer I could accept. An answer that didn't crush my ego. An answer that didn't scare me. An answer that didn't make me think something was really, really wrong with me.

I wasn't ready to be completely honest with myself about why my marriage was falling apart, either. I blamed it on the stress of living in Miami, which gave me an excuse to suggest we move back to Portland. The case I made to Gina: The pace was much slower there and as much as I felt loved and appreciated in Miami, no city had embraced me the way Portland did. Our best times as a couple, I argued, had all been on the West Coast, in Sacramento and Portland.

The real reason I wanted us to move back there? Miami is full of good-looking, super-fit dudes, including one particular Zumba director I suspected was trying to seduce Gina. It was hard for me to trust her because of all the bullshit I had done; now that she was growing in popularity and I was feeling more insecure about the way I looked, I suspected her of doing what I did when I was a hot ticket. Although I didn't have any hard proof, a combination of how I was feeling about myself and her growing success as a dance and fitness instructor was enough. I have a pretty good imagination. The moves in the dance she taught, Zumba, are very suggestive. That's all I needed. (Although my worst fear did eventually turn out to be more than my imagination.)

Looking back, it's clear Gina still wanted our marriage to work, too, because she agreed to the move even though she had grown to like Miami. It didn't help, though, because Bitter, Pill-Popping Brian came with us. To escape, Gina threw herself into her Zumba career, flying all over the world to teach classes—without me. I wanted her to ask me to go with her and she never did. I knew something had permanently changed when I invited her to join me on a surf trip to Costa Rica and she opted to stay home. She would later tell me that my cheating and depressed couch-potato act didn't end it for her; it was how I failed to support her new-found passion the way she had supported mine.

Two positive things did happen once we were back in the Northwest: the Trail Blazers invited me to appear at a game with a few other ex-players and I found the guts to see another neurologist.

Or maybe it wasn't guts, so much as the fact that my desire to know the truth had finally become stronger than my fear of what that truth might be. It was getting harder and harder to pretend I was just dealing with normal stress or depression. The skin tremor had progressed into a jiggling hand and wiggly forearm. Back in Portland, I started coaching my son's basketball team, but I stopped because I didn't know what to tell the kids when my hand would start shaking for no particular reason. I'd try to disguise it by dribbling a basketball, but I could tell by the looks on their faces they weren't buying it. I didn't want to lie to them and I wasn't ready to tell them the truth, so I quit. But if I was afraid of what a handful of 12-year-old boys might think, how was I going to stand in an arena at center court, surrounded by 20,000 fans? How was I going to prevent my hand from doing its thing in front of all of them?

I had considered going into broadcasting as a post-playing career and the Blazers were willing to give me a shot, but I put off their invitations to be part of the team broadcasts and make other public appearances as a team ambassador because I didn't want anyone to see my tremor or ask questions about it. But the thought of once again standing on the court with some former Blazers that I respected, Jerome Kersey and Chris Dudley, to re-live some of the best moments of my life, was more powerful than the fear of public embarrassment. There was also the reason why the team had invited us back: to honor Kevin Duckworth, a gentle giant who had died unexpectedly three months earlier of a heart attack. My NBA career overlapped with Duck's by a few years, but he had moved on from Portland by the time I entered the league and he retired the year before I signed with the Blazers.

It didn't matter that we hadn't played together or never even met; that we had both been Blazers was enough. Plenty of sports teams like to portray themselves as families, but with the Blazers it's the real deal; the fans expect it. Once you've worn that red, black, and white uniform, the organization will give you every opportunity to remain a part of it.

Like me, Duck had moved back to Portland after he retired and, like me, the team had welcomed him back into the fold. He was a midwestern boy, too—from Chicago—but he had adapted an Oregonian lifestyle. He not only hunted and fished but learned to make wooden furniture and became part of the area's arts-and-crafts circuit. (That must have been quite a sight, a 7-foot, 300-pound woodworker roaming the Oregon small-town fairs.) He was on a 19-city tour around the state, drumming up support for the team, when they found him one morning in his hotel room, dead of a heart attack.

Blazers fans have a special place in their hearts for anyone who shows they care about their team as much as they do and Duck did that and more in the 1990 playoffs. Their joy over the team advancing past the first round by beating the Dallas Mavericks that year was tempered by news that they would move on without Duck, who had broken his right hand in the final game against the Mavericks and was ruled out for the remainder of the season. That meant facing the San Antonio Spurs and their Hall of Fame center, David Robinson, without the Blazers' starting center, forcing an array of power forwards—Buck Williams, Kersey, and Cliff Robinson—to take up the slack.

Duck dutifully sat on the bench in a suit with the white club of a cast on his right hand as the two teams split the first six games, the home team winning every time. But after watching the Spurs run away with a decisive Game 6 win in San Antonio, and the decisive seventh game scheduled for Portland's Memorial Coliseum two days later, Duck sawed off his cast—against doctor's orders—and suited up. I can tell you firsthand that no NBA team has louder, more supportive fans than the Blazers, but the roar of the Memorial Coliseum crowd that afternoon shook the building when Duck jogged out of the tunnel and onto the court for warm-ups. (I would feel that same feeling about 10 years later in the Rose Garden.) With Duck putting his big body on Robinson and the crowd inspiring second and third efforts on every possession, Williams, Kersey, and Clyde Drexler were all free to snare double-digit rebounds. That resulted in the Blazers beating the Spurs in a style I could appreciate—out-rebounding them 60–48—for a three-point win.

Duck didn't miss another game. The Blazers beat the Phoenix Suns in six games in the Western Conference finals to reach the NBA Finals for only the second time in franchise history. That's where the party ended, with the defending champion Detroit Pistons, led by Hall of Fame guard Isiah Thomas, winning in five games. Two years later, Duck and the rest of the Blazers would make it back to the Finals only to run in to another defending champion with a Hall of Fame guard, Michael Jordan, and lose in six games. But none of that changed how Blazers' fans felt about Duck and the risk he took on their behalf.

I earned my place with Blazers fans by showing no regard for my personal well-being to help the team advance in the playoffs as well. My time came in 1999, taking an elbow in the head from Utah Jazz Hall of Famer Karl Malone in Game 5 of the Western Conference semifinals. Stepping up and going nose to nose with Karl while blood streamed down my face had the fans in a frenzy when we returned to Portland for Game 6 and we rode their energy to a series-ending win.

But they last saw me in a Blazers' uniform at the peak of my physical powers, which is what terrified me about being seen at the tribute for Duck all these years later. What would they make of this Brian Grant: out of the league, overweight, with a left hand fluttering like a butterfly for no apparent reason?

Even worse, what would my former teammates say? They knew I wasn't the most talented cat, but their respect for how hard I worked meant everything to me. Now I imagined seeing something in their eyes that would hit me harder than if they outright avoided me: pity.

For whatever reason, this time I refused to let my fear and pride get the best of me. I wore a white t-shirt, baggy jeans, a long-sleeved button-down dress shirt and a dark blazer, the better to hide my chunky body. It was a typically chilly fall day in Portland, but I sweated through damn near all of it out of pure nervousness well before halftime. And, of course, the tremor in my hand started up. I played it off as nerves to anyone who asked or even just looked my way. As we waited to walk out onto the court, I confided the truth to Jerome, or at least the truth as I saw it. "I've got this tremor, Romeo," I told him, "but I don't know why."

Kersey was one of the most caring human beings I've ever known. A smile and a pat on the back from Jerome made me feel better, or at least good enough to go through with it. "You'll be alright, big fella," he assured me.

Of course, the rush of standing at center court under the bright lights with all eyes on me again sent my jiggling hand into overdrive. I imagined everyone in the building could see it, so I clasped my hands together, but that set off a chain reaction. Now my shoulders, legs, even my head were twitching and bobbing. When I later saw video footage of that night it was barely noticeable, but that's not how it felt standing out there under those bright lights, all those rows of faces staring down at me from the stands. It felt as if I were doing an involuntary jig. I half expected to wake up the next morning and find a story in *The Oregonian* with a headline, "WHAT'S WRONG WITH BRIAN GRANT?"

There was no such headline or story, of course, but that night convinced me it was time to find out once and for all what I had. A nationally renowned neurologist, Dr. John Nutt, happened to call Portland home and held a teaching residency at the Oregon and Health Sciences University (OHSU). I called and made an appointment to see him.

It was a typical dreary, wet Northwest day when I went in to see Dr. Nutt. Gina was out of town on one of her Zumba tours, so I went in by myself. He checked my weight, tested my reflexes and my balance, and then gave it to me straight: in his opinion, there was no question that I had young onset Parkinson's.

I looked out the rain-streaked window, then down at my lap. "Your scale has to be broken, because there is no way I weigh that much," I said. We both laughed.

It was either laugh or cry and I decided to go with the first one, because I had done enough research at that point to understand his diagnosis meant living a long, healthy life was not in the cards for me.

It's human instinct, though, to cling to the hope that somehow a doctor delivering bad news is wrong, to think of all the stories of people who were misdiagnosed. As a pro athlete, I'd also become accustomed to believing my body could overcome issues the average person's couldn't; I wouldn't have lasted very long in the NBA if it didn't. Dr. Nutt sensed that I might need more convincing. "We can do something to further prove the diagnosis," he said. His recommendation was to go down to UCLA's medical center, where extensive research on Parkinson's has been done, and undergo a test called a dopamine block scan.

I did just that. In very simple terms, dopamine is the missing ingredient at the root of Parkinson's and its symptoms. The test at UCLA consisted of taking some pills that would block any dopamine from getting to my brain so they could take a snapshot of how much dopamine my brain contained in a given moment. Two hours after taking the pills, they had me lie down on a table and strapped my head to it so I couldn't move. Then they slid me inside a device that resembled an open-ended MRI machine. (I'd been in a few of those for my various injuries.) The test lasted another two hours.

Then they sent me home and said they'd call me with the results.

Life went on while I waited. I wasn't the only one in my family dealing with health issues. My aunt Jackie, who lived back in Ohio, had developed breast cancer and needed a mastectomy. I flew back to be with her and the rest of the family at the hospital in Columbus where she was having the surgery. Right after they wheeled her gurney into the operating room, my phone rang. It was a UCLA medical technician.

"Your scan is consistent with young onset Parkinson's," he said. Dr. Nutt, who called right after the technician, would later show me a scan of a normal brain next to mine. The normal one shows all these areas lit up with dopamine like a Christmas tree. Mine was more like Charlie Brown's tree—the gray outline of my brain interrupted by a bright spot here and there.

Catching Karl Malone's elbow in the head was nothing compared to hearing the test results. I hung up and started crying. My family assumed it was because of Aunt Jackie.

"She's going to be alright," they assured me.

"I know she's going to be alright," I said. "It's not that." I wiped away my tears and took a deep breath.

"I just got diagnosed with Parkinson's."

Since that day, I've reflected on how or why I got it. Although brain trauma can be a cause (Ali's is attributed to all the punches to the head he took, particularly late in his career), I don't think I took one too many elbows to the head from Karl or anyone else. My family has since reflected on the family history and someone recalled my great grandfather's brother had a tic of some sort. That's what they probably would've called it back then, "a tic." But it wasn't documented or diagnosed.

Looking back, I was lucky to get the call when I did. One, I was surrounded by family and friends. Two, I could focus on Aunt Jackie and her condition, which was of more immediate concern. But when I laid down that night, and for a lot of nights after that, my mind ran in a million different directions with what this meant. There was only one thing I knew for sure: Philippe had been right.

With that came another reality. The wiring that I had relied on to run faster and play harder to compete against players bigger and stronger than me was now misfiring. My greatest source of pride and confidence, gone. Forget going up against NBA players—my motor skills were so suspect I couldn't trust myself to play in a pick-up game at the Y. In two years I had gone from elite athlete to broken-down jock to someone with misfiring basic motor skills. I was 36 years old and suddenly aware of Father Time staring at me, tapping his watch. And the ticking was all I could hear.

chapter 2
Tough Love

You can find the name "Grant" all over my hometown of Georgetown, Ohio. The street I grew up on is Grant Avenue. There's a Grant museum, a Grant schoolhouse, and a historical plaque with the Grant name on it.

None of that has anything to do with me.

It just so happens another Grant was born a few doors down and 150 years earlier: Ulysses. You might've heard of him—he went on to win the American Civil War as the Union Army general and then became the 18th president of the United States. Most of the houses are not in very good shape on Grant Avenue, but Ulysses' childhood two-story red-brick house has been restored and preserved as a historic landmark. There's a big iron sign with his face on it and a paragraph about his accomplishments.

As a Black kid, though, having the same last name as ol' Ulysses didn't mean shit. He wasn't much more than a White dude with a beard from a long time before I came along; it was only after I read about him in history class that growing up on the same street meant anything. I don't think it ever crossed anyone's mind other than my mom's that we might be related. She's big into genealogy and figured out we weren't connected. (I still wound up with the nickname "The General" when I reached the NBA.)

What stuck with me is how, when the subject did come up, White folk in Georgetown would express their opinion. "He wouldn't be related to you people," is how they'd say it.

We moved around a lot; we even lived in two different places on Grant Avenue. There's a trailer park at the end of the street and that's where my mom, dad, and brother first lived before renting the white clapboard house across the street. There's also a horse farm there that I used to work at as a kid. There was nobody around to enforce child labor laws, apparently, because I remember mucking stalls and helping take care of the horses from 6:00 AM to 6:00 PM. The pay? Getting a ride on one of the horses now and then. I didn't know any other kids who got to ride a horse, though, so I actually thought I was the one getting over.

While Ulysses' house is a lot older than mine, it is in much better shape. Last time I was there my old house was in need of a paint job or at least a power wash, for sure. There used to be trees out front; once upon a time my younger brother, Brandon, climbed up into one of them to sneak a cigarette. My mom smelled the smoke, walked outside, and told him to put the cigarette out and come down out of the tree before she beat his ass. Brandon looked at her, took a big drag, and let the smoke slowly waft out of his mouth. My mom could be tough, but the shock of Brandon being that defiant right to her face made her laugh.

Someone cut the trees down, making it easier to see that the wooden front porch is built directly over the original concrete steps that led up to the front door. It was like that when we lived there; I guess whoever built the porch just didn't want to go to the trouble of jackhammering out the old steps. Sounds funky, right? Trust me, it looks funky. At least now it does. Back then? It was just home.

There's a lot of that new and old jammed together around Georgetown. It's as if everyone wants what's new but is reluctant to let go of the past. Old Ford trucks with their rusty hoods propped open sit in front yards, the driveways reserved for shiny Honda SUVs. Rather than tear down the old high school, it has been converted into a store with neon signs hung in the classroom windows. I suppose it's in the water—I did something similar after I signed my first NBA contract. I bought 12 acres in Georgetown and built my parents a new house farther back on the property but kept the original old house near the street and gave it to one of my sisters.

Some of that is because Georgetown sits in the middle of nowhere, so there's no drive-through traffic or reason for anyone who isn't already connected to the place to invest in it. We had two traffic lights when I was growing up there and they've now added a third; that's about it for growth.

There has been one other change since I left—signs along the country roads leading into town that read, "Georgetown, OH, Hometown of NBA Basketball Star Brian Grant." They're not particularly big; you have to be looking for one to see it and the one on the main road into town is no longer there. If that sounds ungrateful, I don't mean to be. My feelings might be colored by what I experienced growing up or the vibe I get going back there now. I've just never felt as if my hometown ever has embraced that I'm from there. I look at how small towns that have produced NBA players use it as a promotional tool and wonder why Georgetown hasn't done that. I don't care about having a big deal made about me, but I'd be happy to help Georgetown attract more business and development.

There's a famous quote about Cincinnati: "When the end of the world comes, I want to be in Cincinnati because it's always 20 years behind the times." It's not clear who said it, but I understand why they did—it's a very conservative place.

It also means Georgetown would be an even better place to be because you'd get at least another 10 years on top of the 20. No one winds up in Georgetown by accident; if you're driving from Cincinnati, you have to cross the river into Kentucky and then back over again to get there—and going south across the river brings up some uneasy feelings for anyone who is Black and knows their history.

The river, in pre–Civil War days, was supposed to be the dividing line for enslaved people looking to escape the South. Get to the Ohio side and you were officially in the North and a free man or woman. That's what makes the stories of Harriet Tubman, a Black woman, so amazing. She crossed over and back countless times, voluntarily risking her life and liberty by returning to the Deep South over and over again to guide Black brothers and sisters to that finish line.

Not that everybody saw the river as any sort of protective barrier. There was money to be made capturing previously enslaved people and returning them to their enslavers in Kentucky and beyond, making the area around Georgetown a hotbed for slave hunters. Even ol' Ulysses' attitude about slavery was complicated, apparently. His dad, Jesse, was an editor at *The Castigator*, a newspaper in Ripley, Ohio, about 13 miles from Georgetown and was against slavery. But as a farmer in Missouri before the war, records show Grant owned a Black man named William Jones and at one point said he'd be cool with slavery still existing after the war; all that mattered to him was that the Union won. Does that help explain why sharing a last name with the man or living on the same street wasn't looked at by family as something that made us special?

The point I'm making is that just because you were a White person who lived north of the river didn't mean you were against slavery or that you considered Black people as equals. People in Georgetown might've been better at keeping their views on the down low, but you can bet seeing Black people as inferior was handed down from generation to generation long after slavery was abolished. I had family that lived over on the Kentucky side of the river in small towns like Maysville and Mays Lick. The lines were drawn clearly over there—as a Black person, you knew exactly where you could and couldn't go. You knew who in the neighborhood belonged to the Klan because they weren't shy about letting you know. But on the Ohio side in Georgetown and Ripley, they were more discreet; they were there, they just weren't as up front about it.

I can remember being surprised by my grandpa being nice to Ohio people we suspected were Klansmen.

"Why you being nice to them?" I asked him one day.

"It doesn't take anything to be nice to them to their faces," he said. "It's what you do when you can't see them."

"What do you mean by that?"

"I know when I walk away I'm a nigger to them. Just because I'm nice to someone doesn't mean I trust them. Never trust no one." He would school me and my cousins on little things like that. Some White dude might walk by looking funny at him and he'd say, "Hey, how you doing?" That's where I picked up the habit of saying hello first when I meet a stranger. It's more than being friendly. It's also a shield.

Black folk in Georgetown only have to look up to be reminded of the area's dark past. Up on the tree-lined ridge looking over the riverbank is a noticeable gap. A house sits in it and is visible from almost every direction. That house belonged to John Rankin, a local minister who was anti-slavery and apparently a disciple of Paul Revere. The way the story is told in Georgetown, when he got word that there were slave hunters on the prowl, he would put two lights in his window as warning to any newly arrived Black people to stay out of sight. One light in the window signaled it was all clear.

Not everybody, though, had the same view of Black people as Rankin. Let's be real, which side of a river someone lives on isn't going to change their attitude about things, especially how they feel about the color of someone's skin. Besides, a lot of the people living in Ohio had migrated there from the South to take manufacturing jobs as the coal mines closed in Appalachia; they were north of the river to work, not to adopt a different view of Black people.

Maybe that's why most Blacks kept it moving, heading up to Detroit or over to Baltimore. Whatever the reason, Georgetown was 96 percent White and 2 percent Black, and the distrust between White and Black people in Georgetown was alive and well when I grew up there.

It might be less pronounced now, but it's still there, bubbling right under the surface. My younger brother, Brandon, was a much better athlete than I was, but I feel as if, instead of trying to help produce another star from the Grant family, small-town politics took over and the attitude was, "Nah, one is enough. Can't have two." It's not something I can prove, it's just something I believe based on what I feel when I go back, even now. Some of it is the number of pick-up trucks with "Trump 2020" bumper stickers and Trump banners hanging on barns and roadside warehouses. Or the time I tried to pull out of a convenience store parking lot and a man in a red SUV pulled up in front of me, blocking my exit route, and gave me that what-are-you-going-to-do-about-it stare. I rolled down my window and he did the same.

I wasn't going to be the instigator, but I was itching for him to say something crazy. For a second he looked as if he was going to oblige, then saw my three oldest sons sitting in the backseat and thought better of it.

"How you doing today?" I asked.

"Just fine," he said. "That's a pretty nice truck you got there."

"Thank you. Yours is pretty nice, too. Is that new?"

"Newer than yours."

I could've asked what he meant by that but I let it go. "Well, you have a nice day now," I said and pulled out and around him.

There are a lot of good people in Georgetown, too, including plenty who were good to us as kids. There have always been a few mixed in who were extra fucking nasty and seemed to feel it was their duty to let you know that you weren't shit. The best way I can describe the town attitude is how the battle lines were drawn at the main local bar. If bikers rolled in and caused trouble, my family and the local White folk would fight the bikers together. If there weren't any outsiders, then the White folk and my family would fight each other. All I knew is I wanted to be something more than just another soldier in the Georgetown bar-fight army.

My first love in sports was football. I started playing for a Pop Warner team in a neighboring town starting in fifth grade, because Georgetown didn't have a team. I was skinny and pretty weak, but I was quick and I wasn't scared to get hit. I played running back, tight end, and linebacker for the Mt. Orab Broncos until I reached eighth grade and they instituted a rule that you had to be a Mt. Orab resident to be eligible. Georgetown was only a 15-minute drive away but it wasn't close enough. I was good enough that the coaches were willing to have me live with them but my mom wasn't having it, so I switched over to Pee Wee basketball just for something to do.

How bad was I? I was taller than all my friends and had long arms and legs but never got picked in our pick-up games. I had 12 or 13 cousins all around the same age and some of them lived in the same apartment complex, the Markley Apartments, which had a basketball court in the parking lot. The girls who lived in the apartments would come out to watch us, so everyone wanted to show off; I never got the chance, though, because I was never on the court.

Uncle John, my mom's older brother, lived in the Markley Apartments at that time, too, and one summer day he came out while I was sitting on his front steps. He looked over at his son Andre and my other cousins on the basketball court and said, "Why aren't you out there playing?"

"Ain't nobody pick me up," I said.

"Well, shit. Hold on a minute." He went back into his apartment and I could hear him rummaging through a bunch of drawers. When he came back out, he had a little booklet on calisthenics in his hands.

"See this right here?" he said, waving the booklet. "You do what I tell you to do. By the time you're in high school, you'll be sitting on the rim. By the time you go to college, you'll be dunking over the backboard. This'll be our secret, just you and me."

I looked up to Uncle John. There wasn't anybody tougher. It was well-known around town that if you saw him wearing combat boots and carrying his nunchuk, watch out—he was going to war. He got into an argument in a bar one time, ran home for his nunchuk and combat boots, and went at it with some dude. That led to a car chase, with my dad and Uncle John the ones being chased. Uncle John came up with the bright idea of jumping out of the car so my dad could drive away. They were supposedly going about 50 miles an hour when he opened the door and rolled out. It skinned him up pretty badly but he somehow came out of it relatively unhurt. As kids, if we walked by a Georgetown bar and someone said something nasty about us or called us niggers, all we had to do was run home and tell Uncle John. He'd gear up and go looking for whoever yelled at us.

When he informed me he was going to become my personal trainer, I naturally said, "Alright."

For the next two or three days, every time I showed up to play and no one picked me, I'd walk over to Uncle John's apartment and he'd pull out the book and we'd go to work. Every once in a while my cousins would look over and see me doing burpees— or whatever they called burpees back then—and push-up hops and skater jumps and make fun of me.

"Look at that dumbass over there doing that shit with Uncle John," they said.

"Never mind them," Uncle John said. "You just stay with it."

Did those couple of days suddenly make me a different player? No, because it wasn't about making me more athletic. What it did is give me reason to believe I was capable of being something special. There are people who see something in you that maybe you don't see. Uncle John was one of those people for me.

Granted, it was just enough to keep me from quitting, because not a whole lot changed that summer. I might've been a little stronger, maybe a little more coordinated, but I still couldn't even make a layup consistently. The only time my cousins would let me play is if some White boys came down to the court and said, "We want to play you Black boys." My cousins would size them up and then say, "Alright, wait here. We have to get Brian."

I guess my cousins didn't take them as serious competition, so they'd run over to my house and get me. A lot of times they'd find me watching a movie with my mom.

"C'mon, B, we need you, man," they'd say, trying not to laugh. "We need you to stand under the rim and block shots."

Half the time I'd tell them, "You have to wait until the movie is over. You're not going to pass me the ball, anyway." I just wasn't that into it. They'd have to beg me to play. My mom had bought a VCR and like any new piece of entertainment, we were kind of obsessed with renting movies, mostly horror ones. I remember a really violent one, *I Spit On Your Grave*. Or *Dune*. My favorite was *Phantasm*. I'd roll over to the court, block a few shots, then come back home, eat cereal, and watch another movie.

My height got me on the ninth-grade team, but two other freshmen just as tall got called up to varsity. My cousins were upset for me, but it confirmed in my mind that I wasn't very good at basketball, especially since I didn't even play all that much on the freshman team. But Uncle John kept on me. Since the best things I could do were block shots and rebound, he showed me how to score on put-backs or making a drop-step move and then laying the ball into the hoop. Everything I knew about basketball I was getting from him because I didn't grow up watching the game on TV or going to games. I didn't even know any basketball lingo.

"Be a garbage man," he said. "Pick up the garbage and put it in the can."

"What's the garbage?" I asked.

"The damn ball!" Uncle John said.

My mom had a ritual at the beginning of the summer, where she'd buy our school clothes for the next year while they were on sale and put them on layaway. She had me measured when we went to try on the clothes. I was 5'10½" tall. When we went to pick up the clothes and none of them fit, they measured me again. I was nearly 6'4". There is no trade-in policy on layaway, so those were the clothes I had to wear for most of the school year. I sometimes tell people I started the trend of kids wearing their pants halfway down their ass because I had no choice but to do that.

The growth spurt left me with big bumps on my knees from Osgood-Schlatters syndrome, which is what kids get when their bones grow faster than their muscles and tendons. I had the same bumps on my elbows. I grew so much that a lot of my classmates, when they first saw me that fall, thought I might be a new student.

"Brian?" they'd ask, squinting up at me.

"Yeah," I'd say, looking down at them, "it's me."

Despite being so much taller, the pain in my joints kept me from playing basketball my sophomore year. At one point my parents took me in to get x-rays at the local hospital and a doctor visiting from Cincinnati looked at them.

"Do you have tall people in your family?" he asked my mom.

"Not really," she said.

"How tall is his dad?"

"Five-six."

"Five-six?" He glanced out at my dad in the waiting area. "That's his dad?"

"Yeah," she said. "Why?"

The doctor held up the x-ray for my mom. "See these growth plates?" he said. "This child is going to be 6'8" or 6'9"."

The pain subsided enough by the end of the year that I could play in pick-up games, and when my junior year started, both my cousin Jermaine and I were looking forward to finally being on the Georgetown varsity squad.

Maybe it was the heat that first day of conditioning on the track. Or maybe it was the White Southern accent. Or maybe I had been listening to a little too much N.W.A. and forgot I wasn't actually DJ Yella. Whatever set me off, my hopes of playing as a junior ended right there. Jermaine and I were running around the track and a brand-new assistant coach from Kentucky, Jerry Underwood, didn't think Jermaine was running fast enough. I didn't think he was running any slower than some of the White dudes and I didn't like how Jerry said it. I told him as much. Jerry was ready to go. "I'm going to get in your face, boy," he said. "I'll put you on your ass."

"Fuck that," I said. "I'm outta here." Jermaine and I left practice. They let us come back the next day but allowed the players to vote if they wanted us back on the team. They all voted no. Another season had ended for me before it started.

I spent the rest of the school year partying my ass off. School night, weekend, it didn't matter—I'd sneak in and out of my bedroom window and drive over to Maysville, Kentucky, an all-Black town, and get drunk or high or both. There were early mornings I'd barely make it back through the window, still tipsy, before my mom came in to wake me up. "You better get your ass up and go to school," she'd say.

I didn't know exactly how disgusted she was with me until a random incident at the end of the school year provided the spark to light up all the frustration she had been carrying. We were driving somewhere, me in the passenger seat, and a commercial for the University of Cincinnati came on the radio. I still remember the tag line: "UC—Attend now!"

A thought came into my head and I casually said it out loud. "I want to go to college," I said.

Boom! My mom slammed on the brakes and my head smacked into the windshield. Hard. Dazed, touching my forehead to see if it was bleeding, I looked over at her. "What did you do that for?" I asked.

She scowled at me. "What did you just say?"

"You just hit my head on the windshield."

"What did you just say?"

"I want—I'm going to college."

That only made her more mad. "You ain't going to no damn college," she spat. "You ain't gonna be shit. Your dad wasn't shit. And you're gonna be just like your dad. You. Ain't. Gonna. Be. Shit."

Nothing could have hit me harder than hearing my mom tell me I'm worthless and always will be. There wasn't a whole lot I could count on in my life up until then, but my mom's love and support was one. Looking back, it might've been just what I needed. I didn't say anything back to her—I knew better than that—but to myself, I thought, *My mom doesn't think I'm going to be shit. Well, mom, I bet you I graduate.*

It took a few more knocks to the head to finally inspire me to make the most of what I could do on the basketball court as well.

I still remember that first day I showed up at the courts with Andre to play and the older guys were eyeing me. I can't remember what came first: getting chucked into the fence or an elbow to the mouth. All I know is they roughed me up every way they knew how while still playing the game. They didn't outright beat me up, they were just so aggressive I couldn't help but catch an elbow to the head or go face-first into the fence or get scraped up tumbling on the asphalt. Every time, every game, it was the same. Fat lip. Black eye. Bloody nose. I invariably went home with one. The guys made no secret of it, either. "Just so you know, it's going to be this way every time," one of them said, without further explanation. It got so bad, some of the other dudes who showed up to play asked, "Why you messin' with him so bad?" Their response: "Shut up or we'll beat your ass, too."

These were not strangers working me over, either. I knew their names—Kent, Bird, Tim. They lived in Ripley, not far from my grandmother's house. They were all older brothers or cousins of the friends I hung out with in Maysville. I wasn't part of their circle, but I had been cool with them my entire life. No beefs. Before I was old enough to have a driver's license and showing up regularly at the courts, they were the ones giving me a ride to go skateboarding or hang out with their younger brothers.

Finally, one day, they came by my house in a black Cadillac Eldorado. "Get your ass in the car," one of them said. "Now!" Gangsta shit. I was scared. We went through a pony-keg drive-thru and ordered four 40-ounce bottles of beer. I did a quick count of who was in the car. One, two… okay, one must be for me! Maybe this wasn't going to be so bad. I was only 17, so technically I wasn't supposed to be drinking, but that obviously hadn't stopped me during the school year.

Then they drove down to a spot by the river and told me to get out. I did and they handed me one of the 40-ouncers. I don't know if they planned it, but they were doing a great job of getting me to yo-yo between thinking I was going to get punked one minute to feeling I was one of them the next.

They let me drink about half of that 40-ouncer but as soon as I set it down they snatched it away. Then they started in on me. Especially Kent.

"You think I like diggin' ditches?" he said. "Why are you hanging out with my younger brothers and those nasty-ass girls they're messin' with over in Maysville? I love 'em but they ain't shit and they ain't goin' to be shit."

All three took a turn. Then one of them got to the point of it all. I might not have been all that impressed with my game, but they saw the same raw potential Uncle John saw—tall, fast, and fearless despite being so skinny and weak. "You're the first one from around here that might have the opportunity to do something and make us all proud and you want to fuck it up," he said. "So we just wanted to bring you down here and let you know every week you come down here, it's going to be the same shit. You can go get your uncle or whoever, but every time you step on that court, you're going to get your ass busted. You're going to go through that fence."

They were true to their word. I finally did tell Uncle John after one particularly rough outing. "Man," I said, "they tried to throw me through that fence."

"What did you do about it?" he asked.

"Nothing."

"Well," he said, "do something about it. If you need me, I'll come down there, but I want you to do something about it first."

The next three times I went down to the courts, it was more of the same. After the third time, my mom saw me walk into the house. I must've looked particularly beat up. She didn't say anything to me, but that wasn't unusual. I hadn't worked my way back into her good graces just yet. Ever since that car ride, I had tried to straighten up. I'd say goodbye to her in the morning before she went off to work but she wouldn't say anything back. I'd clean the house before she got home and I even got a job at McDonald's—"Yes, ma'am, may I take your order, please?"—but she knew I still spent most of my paycheck chasing girls and getting drunk or high.

Apparently, though, after that third time, she called Kent, Bird, and Tim and cursed them all out. "All of us got a call," Kent told me later. She told us, 'I see his face messed up like that again, it's your asses.'"

I didn't know about my mom getting involved when Andre asked me if I was going back to the Ripley courts for a fourth round. All I knew is that the older guys saw something in me and were going to beat it out of me, if necessary.

"You going back?" Andre asked. Even though he wasn't taking the abuse, it wasn't easy for him to see it happen—and he wasn't anywhere big enough to do something about it.

"Sure am."

"Damn. Alright, I'm going, too, then. I got your back."

Whether it was Andre's support, the older guys letting up a little bit, or understanding why I was getting knocked around, but the first time I got the ball and someone fouled me, I got mad, jumped up, and tried to dunk it. Which I did, barely.

No one was more surprised than me. I had never tried that before. Realizing that I could actually get up high enough to throw it down triggered something in me. I decided in that moment, "You know what? Fuck it. I'm going to do that every time I get the ball."

Next time down the court I went up, another dude went up with me, and I dunked it on him. It was like I'd discovered a super power I didn't know I had. I was still skinny, you could still blow on me and I'd fall over, but for some reason once I got it in my head that I was going to dunk the ball, no one could stop me. As the game went on, it dawned on me: *You are putting it on these cats!*

I sat out a game. When I went back on the court, I noticed that the guys who usually shot around on the other court stopped and were lining up along the fence. It seemed like a few more people had showed up, too. They weren't there to play but just to watch. Word travels fast in a small town and the word was out: "Brian Grant is down at Ripley dunking on people!"

When I went up for that first dunk, it was without knowing if I could actually do it. I surprised myself. Every time I jumped after that, I found myself getting up even higher. This, as it turned out, was why I had been getting beat up. I always assumed Kent, Tim, and Bird had decided to do it on their own. It wasn't until after I retired from the NBA that I found out who put them up to it: Uncle John.

"He's soft," he told them. "Toughen him up. Bloody him up. Rack him." He believed at some point I'd get mad and it would awaken the sleeping beast in me.

No one could say Uncle John's plan didn't work. Suddenly I had a name on the courts in Ripley. It might not sound like much, but it meant a lot to me, someone who'd never had a reputation for anything positive. For a lot of high school athletes, the dream of being recognized is seeing your name in the local newspaper as the "Athlete of the Week." But in places like Ripley or Georgetown, it's more about making a name for yourself in the streets.

The Kings of the Court at that time were the Chamberlain brothers. They lived in Maysville but were considered the best pick-up players in the entire area. I remember watching them in awe when I was younger. They were both around 6'5", not crazy tall, but super strong and athletic. If they weren't dunking on dudes on offense they were at the other end swatting their shots across the court. They owned the paint in any game they played and weren't afraid to tell you.

Word got to Maysville about what I had been doing in Ripley, so one afternoon a caravan of nearly a dozen cars rolled down through that thick, Midwestern summer humidity with the Chamberlain brothers leading the way. Now that I showed I could throw it down, the older guys were happy to have me on their squad. It was Ripley vs. Maysville, pick-up division. Street ball beefs between towns can be as heated as any high school rivalry, with a higher probability of somebody swinging on somebody or running to their car to get a gun. People climbed up on the fence to watch the action on the court and stay clear of the beefs around it.

We not only beat the Maysville boys that day, I dunked on one of the Chamberlain brothers. He was pissed, too! I'm sure if he reads this he'll say, "He didn't dunk on me! Tell me he didn't talk about that!" Street pride runs deep. There's no reason for me to lie. I dunked on his ass.

That was my coming-out party. From that moment on I was no longer Brian the Fuckup but Brian Who Dunked on Tom Chamberlain. The Ripley courts were mine. The older dudes went from slamming me around to having my back if anybody stepped to me. It might not sound like much, but when you've been told you're not shit pretty much your whole life—even by your mom—and all of a sudden you get that moment where you can say, "I am something, I *am* the shit," it's pretty powerful.

Small-town honors are different. Later that summer I got invited to play in Maysville on a court known as the Dirt Bowl. It only had one basket, attached to the side of a building, and the court was only big enough to play three-on-three. It doesn't sound like much and it didn't look like much, to be honest, but it was a special place. It was out of the way, down a little alley near the train tracks—the kind of place you wouldn't know even existed if you weren't a local. People would spend all day down there, barbecuing on the side, but with the court only able to hold six players at a time, you had to be invited to play on weekends. I was, later that summer, and held my own. When it came to outdoor hoops, I had risen through the ranks. Now it was time to find out what I could do on the indoor court at Georgetown High. I was a senior, so this was my last chance and I was determined not to fuck it up.

A few timely breaks helped. The first came when the long-time boys' varsity basketball coach, Bennie Carroll, left for a job at his high school alma mater in Kentucky. I don't know if he would've ever let me on the team if he had stayed. That would've been it, then—everything the townsfolk whispered about me likely would've come true: *He's nothing. He's a troublemaker.*

Carroll, though, unexpectedly left and a guy named Tim Chadwell, who had played and graduated from Xavier University in Cincinnati, took over.

I was committed to proving my mom wrong about my grades and everybody else about what I could do on a basketball court. But two weeks into the new school year I found myself fighting for the chance to play all over again.

The final bell for the day had just rung. My mom had let me drive her car to school that day and Jermaine and me were headed to the student parking lot to get in it and go home. We had just turned a hallway corner when a White kid in glasses hit me with his shoulder, knocking the books out of my hand. I didn't know if it was on purpose or by accident, but he was accompanied by a couple of friends. They were the kind of White boys I liked to jokingly refer to as Future Farmers of America—the kind that were always looking to prove how tough they were. Remember,

Georgetown was 98 percent White, 2 percent Black. I didn't want any trouble, so I let it go and went about picking up my books. I had learned to pick my battles and this one just wasn't worth it.

Jermaine, though, wasn't thinking that way. "You're just going to let him knock your books out of your hand like that and not do anything?" he asked.

"Ah, shit," I said, more to myself than anyone else. I've never been one to start a fight. I'm not even an Old Testament eye-for-eye guy, but question my toughness and we've got a problem. Something sparks up in me and good-natured, mild-mannered Brian Grant can get pretty nasty.

I also knew Jermaine would tell all our cousins that I got punked by some White kid in glasses and didn't do anything about it and I would never hear the end of it. So I turned to the kid with the glasses and said, "Excuse you."

He had an angry squint. "What did you say?"

"I said, 'Excuse you.'"

"I'm not going to say 'Excuse me' to no nigger," he sneered.

All the sideways dirty looks and subtle ways I'd felt disrespected by the Georgetown White folk united like nails to a magnet. Underneath the desire to make him regret what he said, though, remained a lingering fear; not of this kid with glasses or his fellow Future Farmers, but of what might happen if I gave in to all that bottled-up anger.

"Excuse you!" I growled through clenched teeth, poking my index finger into his forehead. I gave his forehead a poke hard enough to put him back on his heels and then turned to pick up my books.

"Look out!" Jermaine yelled.

The kid threw his books on the ground. "Come here, nigger," he said. "I'm going to knock you out!"

I sidestepped him several times while I tried to reason with him. "Hey, I don't want to fight," I said. "I don't…" The superior look in his eye made me snap. Maybe I understood that he wasn't going to take no for an answer. Maybe I was finally done turning the other cheek. I swung and hit him right between the eyes, breaking his metal-rim glasses. He fell back, blood gushing from both eyes as I got in a few more shots before a teacher came running down the hallway and Jermaine and I bolted for the parking lot.

The teacher caught up to us before we could pull away. Jay was the name of the kid I'd beat up. "Brian, you gonna tell me what happened with you and Jay?"

All I could think to say was, "You better not get in my way." I wasn't going to fight a teacher but I didn't know what to do.

"Well, I am going to get in your way," the teacher said, dragging me out of the car. Jermaine tried to tell him to stop. I was just surprised how he was manhandling me because I was so much bigger than he was. Old man strength, I guess. He took me to the principal's office, where the principal said, "You're done. We're expelling you. We don't want you in this school anymore."

In one way I was lucky and in another I wasn't. The lucky part: despite cutting both his eyelids, I didn't do any damage to his eyesight. The unlucky part: the kid still had to go to the hospital to get patched up.

One other not-so-lucky part: he happened to be the son of the county commissioner.

The principal called in both my mom and the boy's dad, who was also one of the biggest pig farmers in the area. My mom was unapologetic.

"I don't teach my son to take no ass-whoopings," she said.

"Did you see his face?" the principal argued, referring to Jay. "He could have gone blind."

My mom didn't back down. "Well, then he shouldn't have called my son a nigger," she said.

"I'm still expelling your son."

"Well, let's see what the NAACP and the local newspapers have to say about that."

The principal might not have cared about how that might look, but the county commissioner did. "I don't want to have any part of this," he said. "My son was wrong. He shouldn't have done it."

The principal wasn't willing to let it go. "You've got to press charges," he told the county commissioner. When the county commissioner waved off that idea, the principal told my mom, "Alright, we won't expel him, but he's suspended for five days. And if you want to take that to the NAACP, go ahead."

My mom had what she wanted. "Alright," she said, and we left.

I found out pretty quickly from my teachers that being suspended for five days was almost as bad as being expelled, as far as being eligible for basketball was concerned. "You're going to have to work hard just to pass my class," one of the teachers told me. "Because every day that you show up you get a certain percentage of points for being there. When you're not there, you lose those points. It's a zero. You're going to have five zeroes to make up."

I thought, "Man, I'm done. There's no way I'm gonna be able to get out of this."

Keep in mind, I already had a reputation for being a poor student and a fuckup, the kind of kid some teachers might think didn't deserve a second chance. I also wasn't about to suddenly get 100 on every test, so I was going to need ways to earn extra credit to cover both my average test scores and make up for the five zeroes. A few teachers were willing to work with me to earn extra credit, but just as many weren't.

Jermaine stayed on me to keep pressing every teacher for ways to lift my grades. I was on my best behavior in class. I crammed for every test and did every extra-credit assignment available. It wasn't because I saw basketball as my ticket to college or anywhere else; those kind of dreams didn't exist in Georgetown. I just wanted to play a year of high school basketball with Jermaine before I had to go work on a farm or in a factory or find some other manual labor job. If you were Black and lived in Georgetown, just landing a job and buying a house was living the dream.

Which is why my dream was to get the hell out of Georgetown.

Two summers before I made my name on the Ripley courts, I sat on my porch on a summer night looking up at the stars and said a prayer. "West End Girls," a song by the Pet Shop Boys, had become one of my favorites, mostly because of the lyrics. It was an early Euro version of rap at that time, inspired by a Grandmaster Flash song called "The Message." It was about "East End boys," or dudes from the poor side of town, living in "a dead-end world" looking to escape by hooking up with higher society "West End girls."

I saw myself as an East End boy stuck in Georgetown. I prayed that night, "Lord, let me go west and meet a beautiful woman and start a family. I'll work as hard as my body will let me if it will make that possible."

The Lord did indeed make it possible. What I did with it is another story.

I don't know what kind of textbooks they use today, but you could find the word "nigger" in the ones used in American History classes at Georgetown High. There were 20 students in the class and I was the only Black one. We had to take turns reading out loud and no one seemed to have a problem saying that word. Every time it was said, though, I felt as if everyone looked at me. I just kept my head down and stared at my book, waiting for the moment to pass.

Mr. Stanley Martt, the American History teacher, was already one of the oldest teachers at the school when he had my dad in his class, so you know he was up there by the time he had me as a student. His approach to teaching was from an earlier era, too. He was the make-you-stand-in-the-corner, rap-your-knuckles-with-a-ruler type teacher. There were a few of us who spent quite some time standing in the corner because he also had a blind spot in his left eye, and we were constantly trying to see what we could get away with by taking advantage of it.

He used phrases like, "I'd be on your ass like a duck on a June bug," which didn't sound like something a teacher should be saying to any student.

All of which made me really nervous when I had my last test with him and I couldn't afford to have more than one wrong answer on it to get the overall grade I needed. I crammed like hell for it, but when Mr. Martt called me up to his desk at the end of class, I had a bad feeling.

"Sit your ass down," he said, motioning to the chair next to his desk. He shook his head. "Son, you can't beat up people every time you get called the 'n' word or you'll be fighting people all your life."

"I know," I said. "I wish I hadn't done it."

He had my test paper in his hands. Ten multiple choice questions. I could see that four of the answers had been marked wrong. "What's this?" he asked.

"I crammed," I said. "I'm not making excuses but I crammed for it."

He pointed to the first one I had wrong. I'd circled D, but looking at it now I knew the answer should've been C. "It's C," I said.

"Why didn't you put that?" he asked, marking it correct. Then he went to the next one I got wrong and pointed to it. I gave him a different answer and he marked it correct. We went through the same routine with the third one.

"Son," he said, "sometimes people give you second chances. You just got yours. You better make the most of it."

I walked out of his classroom crying. Jermaine was waiting for me in the hallway. When he saw my tears he presumed the worst.

"Oh, man," he moaned. "You can't play."

"Dude," I said. "Guess what happened." I told him exactly what Mr. Martt did and then made him promise he wouldn't tell anyone else. I didn't want to get Mr. Martt in trouble. The only other person I told was my mom. I imagined if one of my classmates found out, they'd tell the principal, who I could see happily making my original test score stand to make me ineligible.

Jermaine couldn't believe Mr. Martt, of all people, would do me that kind of favor. "Whaaaat?" Jermaine shrieked. "Mr. Martt did that?" Then it kicked in what all this meant. "You get to play!"

Mr. Martt's second chance led to another one. Chadwell, the new varsity coach, met with Jermaine and me.

"Boys, everything I've heard about you and everything everyone has said is that I should not take a chance on you," he said. "But I'm here to tell you I don't care what they say. I don't care what you've done. I'm going to judge you from here on out. Is that fair?"

Jermaine and I looked at each other and nodded. "That's fair," we said.

"Alright, good. You'll be on my team this year."

We had been dreaming of wearing legit uniforms and playing in that Georgetown High gym in front of our families since we were kids playing sock ball with a bent coat hanger hooked over a door frame for a hoop—and we already knew exactly what we were going to do for the first play of the first game. Coach Chadwell might not have known, but we did.

Our plan—Jermaine and mine—was to bring that Ripley Courts swagger to the Georgetown High gym. After a summer of dunking on grown men where only a busted lip or being thrown into the fence warranted a foul, playing against kids my age with refs blowing the whistle for an incidental bump promised to be a snap. We were ready to shock the world, or at least our small part of it.

We had secretly been planning that first play for months. I would jump center and tip the ball to the left side of the floor toward our basket. Jermaine would already be breaking that direction, anticipating that I'd win the tip; if I was jumping high enough to dunk on asphalt courts, what were the chances anyone could out-jump me on a relatively bouncier hardwood floor? As soon as I landed I'd take off on a dead sprint down the right side of the floor, trusting that Jermaine would be first to the ball. As soon as I cut toward the basket, Jermaine would then throw a lob for me to slam home.

Not everything works out as you plan it. My life offers all the proof you need of that. But this was one time when it worked out exactly as we planned it. Maybe even better. Because what we hadn't anticipated was the reaction.

Since I had been dunking all summer on outdoor courts, the idea of throwing one down in a gym didn't feel like a ground-breaking event. There was a player a few years older than us who we all admired because he could dunk, and Georgetown fans would get excited when he did, but some dunks are just more dramatic than others. What I had not taken into account is that pretty much everyone in the gym had never seen me play, much less dunk. I'm sure to a lot of them I was still Brian the Fuckup.

Not to toot my own horn, but there is something different about the way I dunk. My jump is quick and I love throwing the ball down just as hard and quick. It's like two explosions, back to back. So when I soared above the rim to catch Jermaine's lob with both hands and then flushed it so hard the entire backboard shuddered, the entire gym went nuts. I guess no one was expecting something that dynamic in the opening seconds of the game from two guys they'd never seen before in a Georgetown uniform. They didn't cheer—they howled. Between the adrenalin of playing in front of the whole school and on a bouncy wooden floor, I did get up pretty high. The howl caught the attention of everyone outside the gym. They poured in through the doors, eager to find out exactly what had happened. The game went on, of course, but at the first stop in play it was clear no one had forgotten how Jermaine and I kicked it off. Our teammates mobbed us and people in the front row were slapping us on the back. It was as if we'd already won the game (which we eventually did).

I took a second to look around and soak it in. People who, just the day before, would've shook their head or turned away if they saw me walking down the street were smiling and clapping for me. It was as if they'd never seen anyone dunk a lob before and maybe they hadn't, at least not the way I did it.

"This," I thought, "is some different shit."

Different shit that became regular shit. The buzz around town about how hard I was dunking prompted all sorts of local businessmen and others to stop by practice, thinking they could just walk in and watch.

You should see Brian Grant throw it down.

Oh, he can dunk now?

Dunk? He's tearing the rim down!

Chadwell kicked them all out, but that only made our games that much more must-see.

No matter how crowded the stands were, though, when my mom and the rest of the family showed up, they'd clear a path through the crowd and find them seats right near center court. The same people that called us niggers and had always looked at us on the street like they didn't trust us were now treating us like royalty.

"This," I said to myself, "is *definitely* some different shit."

The downside to becoming a big deal was my relationship with my dad and my cousins. It started with that initial growth spurt and only got worse when I started to blow up as a basketball player. My cousins struggled accepting that I wasn't the weak, awkward Brian who'd rather be home watching movies with his mom that they'd grown up with; and I hadn't forgotten how, game after game, they wouldn't pick me to play. They wanted to put me back in my place and I had no interest in being put back there, prompting a lot of fights.

My dad, meanwhile, was constantly being teased by my uncles about being so much shorter than me. He'd get pissed and want to take it out on me. I spent most of my high school years staying away from him.

Not that Jermaine and I ever imagined our sudden small-town fame leading to anything. We figured that eventually it would all go back to the way it was before. Nothing really changes in places like Georgetown. We just wanted to enjoy the wild attention for however long we could, piling up the mental snapshots and stories to share when it was all over so we'd have something to talk about while we were picking tobacco or loading trucks or whatever we'd end up doing to afford a car and a place to live and a good time over in Maysville.

A couple of weeks into the season, Chadwell did let a man wearing a Xavier pullover in to watch our practice. We were about halfway through when the stranger walked in, caught about 10 minutes, and then disappeared into the coach's office with Chadwell for 20 minutes.

After the stranger left, Chadwell called me in to see him.

"Son, where do you want to go to school?" he asked.

I couldn't imagine why he was asking. I didn't really know anything about schools in general or basketball schools in particular, but I'd heard my cousin mention Syracuse and Georgetown, so that's what I told Chadwell.

"Okay, I'll call them for you. Because that was Dino Gaudio from Xavier. They want you. And if a school like that wants you, a lot of others would, too."

Apparently, someone had been anonymously calling the Xavier basketball office and telling them they had to come check out this senior power forward at Georgetown High. As a small school in Division IV, college scouts never attended our games. Whether it was out of curiosity or just a desire to tell the anonymous caller they'd seen me so they could stop calling—I never found out who it might have been—Xavier head coach Pete Gillen had finally sent an assistant, Gaudio, to see me play. Or, more accurately, to see me practice. It tells you just how genuinely interested Xavier was that it wasn't even willing to spend two bucks to get into a game.

"Go out there, buy yourself a country biscuit, and call it a day," I imagined Gillen telling Gaudio.

That one practice was enough for Gaudio.

"How many people know about this kid?" he asked Coach Chadwell.

"Nobody," he said.

"Let's keep it that way," Gaudio said.

It didn't quite stay that way. Youngstown State made me an offer and several NAIA schools were interested as well. I also got invited to visit the University of Cincinnati by then-coach Bob Huggins. Whether it was that radio jingle or the down-and-dirty way the Bearcats played, I liked the idea of going to UC.

Chadwell went with me and almost right from the start something felt off. Huggins met us, along with another recruit, but then took the other recruit on a tour and handed me and Chadwell off to an assistant coach. When we went to the game, the other recruit sat on the UC bench while Chadwell and I were given seats way off in a corner.

"There ain't no damn way you're going here," Chadwell said. I was disappointed, but I agreed. (Huggins told me many years later that he didn't put much effort into recruiting me because he had been told I wouldn't have the requisite SAT scores to get admitted. It's hard for me to believe that was the reason because Huggy Bear wasn't exactly known for recruiting scholars—UC eventually let him go because only about 30 percent of his players graduated while he was there.)

At that point, I still wasn't convinced I'd actually become a Musketeer, either. Georgetown only lost two regular-season games all year—one to a team from a higher division and one where I didn't play because of the flu—but we didn't have anyone from our team picked to the Division IV All-Ohio team.

Keep in mind, Division IV was the lowest division in Ohio boys' basketball and they selected six players to the first team, six to the second team, five to the third team, and then had an additional "special mention" group where they listed *21* players. You'd think having that kind of record without a single player considered All-State-worthy would earn Chadwell recognition as Coach of the Year, but he didn't get any shine, either. I kind of get it: the teams are selected by a panel of sportswriters and broadcasters and the only time I saw one of the local TV crews at one of our games was when we played the higher division team. If I was really on the radar of Division I programs, shouldn't I be somewhere among the top 38 Division IV high school players in my state?

Xavier didn't exactly close the deal until the last minute, either. After we lost in the district semifinals and missed our chance to go to state, Gillen and Gaudio approached me outside the locker room. "We have one scholarship left," he said. "It's between you and a kid from Mt. Healthy. It's yours if you want it."

I didn't waste a second. "I'll take it," I said.

"Did you hear that, Dino?" Gillen asked, turning to his assistant. "Brian has verbally committed to Xavier."

I nodded and repeated what he said, the way you do when you're getting married and the minister feeds you your lines. Or when you're in a court room and you pledge an oath. Instead of "I solemnly swear…" I said, "I verbally commit."

Gaudio shook my hand. "Welcome to Xavier," he said. "Alright, then. You guys take it easy."

And that was pretty much it. There wasn't much more fanfare than that. But in Georgetown it was a big deal. Xavier had just upset Georgetown in the NCAA tournament to advance to the Sweet 16 and everyone in the area knew their two stars—and future NBA players—Tyrone Hill and Derek Strong, especially after they took down Georgetown's future NBA stars, Alonzo Mourning and Dikembe Mutombo. At school the next day, the entire school heard over the P.A. system as part of the morning announcements: "…And we want to congratulate Brian Grant, who has committed to Xavier University!"

There was also a local businessman who bought everyone on the team these yellow jackets with a big letter "G" on them. If you had one of those, you were the shit. The same businessman gave me a job after the season making deliveries to the local mom-and-pop convenience stores. It was a favor that allowed me to have something in my pocket when I went to Xavier, but he made sure he was getting his money's worth. I got paid minimum wage and he worked my ass hard. I'd come home exhausted. His brother saw me loading all these boxes and finally stepped in and said that I'd be working for him, instead. I didn't expect anything to be all that different, but I learned otherwise pretty quickly. After my first job, cleaning out the gutters at his house, he handed me a $100 bill. Sometimes he'd have me work for an hour or so and then say, "Let's take the boat down to the river," and we'd chill the rest of the afternoon, riding around on his boat on the Ohio.

I never thought life would be that good, or that a White person from Georgetown would be that nice to me. I'd gone from being seen as a troublemaker to a small-town hero. I still think about Mr. Martt, more than anybody else, to this day. If it weren't for his decision to let me re-take that test until I had the score I needed, I wouldn't have been eligible to play, which means the anonymous caller would've had no reason to call the Xavier basketball office. My life would've played out in a whole different way. I might've never made it out of Georgetown. I still wish Mr. Martt hadn't made us read the word "nigger" out loud in class, but I'm happy to call us even.

Before the summer was out, though, I would be reminded more than once that there were still plenty of skeptics out there waiting for me to fall on my face. There were times I happened to be one of them.

chapter 3
I Don't Belong Here

Despite not being an All-State selection, I was invited to play in a postseason all-star game called the Ohio North-South Game. It's actually two games, the first being a showcase of players from the top two high school divisions and the second being for the lower two. One guess as to which game the skinny kid from Georgetown High was invited. Going to Xavier on a full ride earned me an invitation, but it wasn't enough to get me out of the "B" game.

Chadwell did his best to convince the organizers I belonged on one of the "A" squads but they thought he was crazy for even suggesting it. A Division IV kid who wasn't All-State—wasn't even All-State *special mention*—in the "A" game? One of my best friends, Tyrice Walker, Ohio's Mr. Basketball and headed to Xavier with me, made a case that I should be in the "A" game with him as well. They didn't believe him either. Granted, they were asking for something extraordinary—it would be like suggesting someone performing community theater deserved a Tony. But did their flat-out refusal give me a little extra fuel? You bet it did.

The "B" game was played first and after getting over some nervousness in the first few minutes, I did what I had been doing all year—grab the rebound on defense, pass it to a guard, beat everybody to the other end, and wait for a lob pass back to smash on someone's head. Everyone seemed stunned that someone that tall—I was 6'7" by then—could be the fastest guy on the court. The "A" game players rolled in during the second half and started pumping me up. "Hey, man, you're real," they said. "You're just throwing that shit down on people."

Gaudio was there, too. "Boy, I don't think Pete knows what he's getting with you," he said. "You are the shit. I can't believe we got you."

Chadwell sidled up to the organizers before the "A" game started with a satisfied smile. "Told you all," he said.

I was pretty quiet back then. Being recognized and praised was something still relatively new and I wasn't sure how to take it. The skeptical, cynical, suspicious part of me thought they were all just blowing smoke, saying what they thought I wanted to hear, so I didn't believe Gaudio reeeeeeally thought all that much of me. Besides, for all my success, some people in

Georgetown still considered it a fluke that I'd made it to college and were certain I wouldn't actually play.

All the freshman players were enrolled in a three-week summer session to get acclimated to college life and take some preliminary classes. They were offering us a head start—or in my case, a chance to catch up. At the start of the three weeks we took a test in each class to find out exactly how prepared we already were. I walked into my math class, I sat down, opened the test booklet, took one look, closed it, and walked out of the class. It was Algebra and although I had earned a C- my senior year at Georgetown in pre-Algebra, I didn't know anything about Algebra.

I was called in by Sister Rose Ann Fleming, who oversees all the academic counseling for the school's athletes.

"So, I hear you walked out of your math class without taking the test," she asked. "How come?"

I was embarrassed but I told her the truth. "I don't know anything about algebra," I said. Another lucky twist of fate. Entrance qualifications for colleges and universities in Ohio were raised a year later. I would not have been eligible to go to Xavier knowing nothing about algebra, which Sister Fleming pointed out to me.

My eyes started to well up with tears. "Maybe I shouldn't be here," I said.

She tilted her head toward me. "Do you want to be here?" she asked softly.

"Yes, absolutely."

"I'll make this promise to you, then," she said. "If you do the work, I'll get you every tool you need—tutors, counselors, study guides—to make sure you stay eligible."

"I'll do the work," I said. "That's my promise to you."

I've heard about top-flight schools where smart students or academic advisers take tests for the student athletes to keep them eligible, but that wasn't happening at Xavier when I was there. You had to do the work, and if you failed, you could go ahead and pack your bags because you were out. Sister Fleming kept her promise and I kept mine, although I had to ratchet down my educational ambition. Signing up for classes is sort of like a bake sale—there are all these tables set up with pamphlets promoting different kinds of classes and careers. Every athlete was accompanied by another student to make sure we enrolled in the appropriate classes. "I'd like to be a lawyer or a doctor," I said.

"Whoa," my guide said. "Those are great majors. But they take up a lot of time and so does basketball. I think you'd be better off getting a degree in something like organizational communications."

Message received. I might've been from a small town with no expectations of ever going to college, but I understood when someone tried to say something without saying it. "Organizational communications it is," I said. I couldn't tell you today exactly what I learned from that major, but it kept me eligible for four years and I graduated with a college degree in it.

Being on campus early also allowed me to be a counselor along with the other incoming freshmen players at a week-long youth basketball camp. Erik Edwards, a 6'8", 250-pound power forward, was the most well-known and highly coveted recruit in our class by far. At this time, AAU basketball had not become the center of the youth basketball universe and the place to be seen if you wanted to go to college. High schools still ruled and Edwards played for a big-time school, Wilmington High in Delaware. The Wilmington Red Devils were invited to play in the Great Florida Shoot-Out, one of the premier pre-Christmas tournaments. Edwards was named an All-American and played in the Dapper Dan Roundball Classic, a national All-Star game for high school players that ended in 2007 but once was as prestigious as today's McDonald's All-American game.

One of the campers approached our table in the cafeteria and asked Erik for an autograph. The camper glanced at me. "Who is that?" he asked.

"Oh, that's Brian," Erik said. "He'll play when I leave after my junior year for the NBA."

The camper looked at me for confirmation. I looked at Erik, surprised by his snap judgment on how our careers at Xavier were going to play out. I could feel the heat rising from my gut to the veins in my neck to the top of my high-top fade.

"That's right," I said to the camper, playing it cool in the moment.

Now, I had no idea if or when I was going to play; for all I knew Edwards was right. But the dismissive way he said it, when I knew he had never seen me play, got me as fired up as being put in the North-South "B" game. Maybe more, because this was personal. He had put me down with me standing right there. I made a mental note to myself: *First chance I get, I'm letting ol' Erik know what happens when you underestimate this Division IV kid from Georgetown.*

Tyrice was at our cafeteria table and took the comment the same way I did. "You motherfuckers might want to stop talking to Brian that way," he warned them. "He be out there ballin'."

Freshmen from all the fall sports were invited to the three-week summer session and paired up randomly as roommates and study partners. Allen Dullin, a tennis player, was my roommate. He knew how quiet I was and, conversely, had heard how the other incoming freshmen basketball players talked when we were together in the cafeteria or study hall. They were very confident and he was worried that it was getting to me. "You know what, BG, your guys are always talking," he said. "Don't worry about it."

He was right about it getting to me—but he was wrong about how. I wasn't worried; I was mad. A couple days after the youth camp ended, a bunch of us on the team got together on the campus outdoor courts to play pick-up. Erik and I, both being 6'8", naturally were matched up against each other.

The first time I got the ball, I dunked over him and stared him down. "What do you got to say now?" I asked.

He came right back at me. "Oh, you wanna talk shit?"

The next time I got the ball I went at him again—and dunked again. "This is where I do my talking," I said. "On the court."

I'm not sure what triggered all that. I had never been good at talking smack. I hadn't watched that much basketball, but I had grown tired of hearing all these other freshmen talking about their games in front of me every day for almost two weeks as if they didn't consider me competition. A piece of advice to all of you out there: Don't think the quiet one in your circle isn't taking in everything. Just because they're not talking doesn't mean they're not listening. Or taking notes on what they've heard. And transforming it into fuel to feed a fire that ends up burning you.

I might've dunked every basket I scored. I didn't say anything when we finally finished. Steve Gentry, an incoming point guard, said it for me: "Man, Brian kicked y'all's ass."

I started scoring a few points off the court as well. In Georgetown, there weren't a lot of Black girls—hell, there weren't a lot of Black people, period. To date a Black girl, you had to drive about 45 minutes either direction just to find one that wasn't somehow related to you. Dating White girls wasn't much easier if you were Black; in and around Georgetown, a White girl would get her ass whupped by her dad if he found out she was dating a Black dude. Her older brothers or sisters were just as likely to come down on her. I did date a few White girls in high school, but they didn't last very long and we had to sneak around the whole time.

As different as Xavier might've been from how I grew up, I didn't have as much trouble adjusting as some of my teammates who were from the inner city or downtown. The five freshmen on the team were required to live in the dorms and they put us together on the first floor of the Westside building. Every Friday, the priest who lived on the second floor, Father LaRocca, would make a big pot of pasta and everyone in the dorm was invited to chow down from 6:00 to 8:00 PM. Then he'd read some scripture, nothing too heavy, and talk about what we could learn from it.

I saw it as a great way to meet students outside the athletic program. For my teammates, though, it was culture shock. They were from all-Black inner-city neighborhoods in places like Chicago and Wilmington, Delaware. Being surrounded by so many White kids made them uncomfortable. One of my teammates in particular was always ready to fight someone over the music they were playing. Having grown up hearing everything from my Georgetown classmates' Van Halen and Aerosmith tapes to my mom's songs by The Carpenters and Bread, I was open to just about anything. One night I was sitting in the dorm room of two regular students, listening to Pink Floyd, when the teammate in question pounded on the door and yelled, "Turn that shit off!"

He was surprised when I opened the door. "What are you doing in there?" he asked.

"Listening to *Dark Side of the Moon*," I said.

"You like that shit?"

"Yeah."

"Okay." He went back down the hall, shaking his head.

My dorm mates introduced me to The Grateful Dead and Steely Dan, among others. I was into all of it.

Nothing racist happened to me on campus, that I can recall, but I always had my radar up. If I went off-campus to the movies or just walked down the street with a White girl, I could feel eyes on me and I could guess with one glance at the face of whoever was staring at me what they were thinking. "That motherfucker," I'd say under my breath and my girlfriend at the time would ask, "What do you mean?"

"You don't see what I see."

I met a girl named Lisa early in my freshman year, and she invited me home to have dinner with her parents. I was nervous. "Are you sure you want to take me to your parents' house?"

"Yeah, my parents are cool," she said. The family was devoted to all things Xavier and apparently had players from the basketball team over for dinner all the time. Michael Davenport, a senior on the team, knew the family well; he'd had dinner at their house, too.

"Is it cool to go over for dinner?" I asked.

"Oh, yeah, they're nice," he said.

Her mom made chicken thighs for dinner and slathered them with Montgomery Inn barbecue sauce, a personal favorite. I might've eaten a half dozen of those thighs. While we ate, Lisa's three younger brothers peppered me with questions. "You going to do good this year?" one of them asked.

"I don't know," I said. "I'm just a freshman."

"Yeah," one of the other two said, "we've never heard of you."

I had to laugh at that. I also found it funny that every time I went over to their house, it just so happened they were having chicken thighs again. What were the odds of that? I suspected I knew why, but I wasn't about to complain. Then one day Lisa brought me home for dinner by surprise. We walked into the kitchen and a big pot of spaghetti was on the stove.

Her mom looked shocked. "Why didn't you tell me you were bringing Brian home?" she asked. "I'll be right back."

She came back 20 minutes later with a grocery bag full of chicken thighs. Lisa was mortified. "Mom! I can't believe you did that!"

"Well, he loves them!" her mom said. She was kind of flustered.

"It's okay," I said. "But I do eat things other than chicken."

There was also a play, *The Foreigner*, put on by Xavier's student theater company while I was there. I don't remember it and I doubt I saw it, but in the yearbook it is described as "a comedy which took a light-hearted look at a serious problem— racism and the prominence of the KKK in the South... The cast and crew were successful; they portrayed their characters to perfection and presented a convincing image of the South. *The Foreigner* provided the viewers with some food for thought and many fits of laughter."

There's a chance the description in the yearbook just didn't strike the right tone, but my life experience to that point made looking at the KKK in a light-hearted way a stretch. Then again, making presumptions about or looking down at a Black boy from the country wasn't limited to White people. There were a healthy number of other Black students on campus, so I decided I'd look for a woman of color to date. One day I walked up to these six Black ladies and said, "Hey, how you doin'?"

They did everything but turn their backs on me. One of them looked at me as if she smelled something bad and said, "Ugh, you sound like you're White and country."

I said, "Excuse me?"

"You sound country and White."

(I would later learn her name was Carol, because my best friend, Tyrice, ended up marrying her.) I hadn't had a whole lot of experience talking to girls of any color in Georgetown—and I knew Georgetown was a lot different than Xavier. I wasn't considered handsome by any stretch; in fact, growing up I was often made fun of for my looks, along with being unusually tall. I was self-conscious about it all. So it took everything I had just to walk up and say hello—and now you're going to tear me down?

So the next week, I ran in to Lisa and said, "How you doin'?" and got a completely different reaction. I never felt fully accepted by either side. I knew the families of the White girls I spent time with were not thrilled about their daughters dating a Black dude. Then, if I was with a White girl going to a movie theater in one of Cincinnati's black neighborhoods, I could feel the sisters staring holes in me, as if I was deserting my kind. I was having none of it, though; I didn't go looking to date a White girl—I did it because she showed interest and the Black girls didn't.

I did date one Black girl in high school. Trina Smith was my best friend growing up and the one Black girl in the area who wasn't somehow related to my family. As a result, she ran through eight of my cousins who at some point called her their girlfriend. There wasn't anything sexual going on with any of them beyond kissing or a little feeling up. We had this thing where we'd cruise town on Friday night and the middle of the backseat was called Piper's Pit. I'd sit on one side and my friend Keith sat on the other. The rules were that if a girl decided to sit between us, we had the time between one stoplight and the next to do whatever we wanted with her. It usually wasn't more than seven to 10 seconds and it might sound funny or perverted but it wasn't more than a grab or a squeeze. It never got out of hand. The girl would be laughing and shouting, "Get to the light! Get to the light!"

One night we were hanging out late, parked off on the side of a country road listening to music, and Trina was sitting next to me. My hand slipped down and brushed her leg. Then she put her hand on my hand and started stroking it. That caught me off guard. I had always liked her but Trina, years earlier, said, "No, you're my best friend. We're in the same grade."

Now, in the back of the car, I stroked her hand even as I said to myself, "This is Trina, my best friend—what the fuck is going on?"

When we started kissing in the backseat, it was so out of character for us that everybody in the car was startled. "What are you all doing?" someone said. "Oh, my God, they're kissing!" someone else said.

I go to school on Monday and Trina won't talk to me. I'm not sure what to think. Did I lose a best friend trying to get a girlfriend? Then one of her girlfriends was dating a guy I was friendly with and she arranged a double date after the Friday basketball game. We went out, some things happened, and suddenly we were boyfriend and girlfriend.

As soon as that became official, Trina became rather possessive. She now distrusted the girls that we'd been hanging out with for years. "Those are our friends," I said.

"I know, but you need to quit talking to them anyway," she said.

"Oh, God," I thought to myself. The relationship lasted about five weeks during my senior year. That was about it when it came to girlfriends in high school.

On the basketball court, Dino Gaudio's belief in what I could be turned out to be right—great judge of talent, that Dino Gaudio. We were scheduled to play the Polish national team in a preseason exhibition when Maurice Brantley, a sophomore guard, missed a class and was held out of the game. Gillen lined us up on the baseline the morning of the game and walked back and forth in front of us, barking in his raspy voice, "Mo got in trouble and now I've got to start a damn freshman," he said, "and I don't want to start a damn freshman." Even though I had been playing well in practice, I thought for sure Erik would get the nod; he was the All-American, after all, and I was the last player to land a scholarship, one rung up from the walk-ons who made the squad.

"Brian, you're starting," Gillen said. My jaw dropped, along with Erik's and everyone else's.

As I sat on the training table getting my ankles taped, I was so nervous I thought I was going to hyperventilate. Tyrice tried to calm me down, but it didn't do much good.

The first play of the game, one of our guys took a shot that skidded off the rim. I went up and grabbed the ball on one side of the rim and my momentum carried me to the other side, where I reverse dunked it. I didn't plan it, it was just an instinctive reaction. The crowd went crazy. That didn't calm me down as much as it channeled my energy. I went from being nervous to excited, realizing in that moment that I was just as capable of crushing dunks in college as I had been in high school.

But I also had a healthy fear that if I ever slipped up and lost that starting spot, I might never get it back. (Mo didn't.) That kept me going hard every game—and kept me in the starting lineup. We had been expected to fall off after losing forwards Tyrone Hill and Derek Strong to the NBA from a team that had gone to the Sweet 16 the year before, even with the Musketeers landing Tyrice and Erik. What they didn't count on was me leading the entire Midwestern Collegiate Conference in rebounding, averaging nearly a rebound a game more than the conference's next best.

We were never ranked among the top teams the entire season, but we won the conference tournament, earning an automatic berth in the NCAA tournament as a 14th seed. No. 3 seed Nebraska tried to out-muscle us and failed, fouling us enough that we outscored them 29–14 in free throws for a huge 89–84 upset. No one took advantage more than I did, scoring nine of my 15 points at the line. I had another solid performance against the 11th-seeded UConn Huskies—16 points, 12 rebounds—but no one else scored in double figures, we missed 14 of 18 three-point attempts, and lost 66–50.

The dip came my sophomore year, after we lost our starting backcourt, Michael Davenport and Jamal Walker. We didn't get a postseason invitation to the NCAA tourney or the NIT.

I found a whole new level of motivation my junior year, when I lost a younger cousin, Junior. We'd had a falling out over a girl and hadn't talked for nearly a year. I finally invited him over to my apartment near campus and told him I loved him and wanted to get past our differences. We settled it by going to a club called Cooter's near the University of Cincinnati campus. We stayed out pretty late and I invited him and my cousin Jermaine to crash at my place, but they said they were good to drive and wanted to get back to Georgetown.

The next morning my mom was blowing up my phone. When I finally called her back, she said, "Junior was in a car accident last night. He's in the hospital. You need to get over here right away."

Junior was riding in a car with his best friend; Jermaine was in the car behind them. Junior's friend fell asleep at the wheel, crossed the center lane, and smashed head-on into an oncoming car. The drivers of both cars escaped any serious injury, but Junior was thrown from the car into a ditch. That's where Jermaine found him when his car pulled up a minute later.

An EMT just happened to be driving down that same two-lane highway and stopped when she saw the wreckage. Junior was having trouble breathing and she helped position his neck to alleviate that until an ambulance arrived.

Junior was in the intensive care unit on a ventilator. The entire family spent the next three days in his room or camped out in the hospital lobby. They finally determined he was brain dead and not coming back. His dad, my Uncle David, and me were in the room when they took him off the machines keeping him alive. His eyes were open and I watched him pass.

It tore me up that we'd spent so much time mad and avoiding each other. It set something off inside me. It happened as we were preparing for the season, and basketball became my outlet for the rage I felt. Any opponent that had the misfortune of being matched up with me faced a maniac seeking revenge against the force out there that had taken my cousin. I already felt indebted to Xavier and Coach Gillen for getting me out of Georgetown; when they came to Georgetown to attend Junior's funeral and mourn with me, I was ready to give everything to see Coach and the Musketeers succeed.

I led the team in scoring and rebounding and won my first of two Conference Player of the Year Awards while we cruised to a 24–6 record and another trip to March Madness. This time we were the ninth seed and knocked off eighth-seeded New Orleans before losing to No. 1 Indiana in Indianapolis inside the RCA Dome, a football stadium that was a field of Hoosier red that night.

My senior year might've broken the cycle but we didn't know how to deal with prosperity. Almost as soon as we climbed into a spot in the national rankings, we'd respond with a loss that dropped us right out of them again. We were ranked 22nd when we upset ol' Bob Huggins and UC, which was nationally ranked 19th at the time, but three nights later we lost to conference rival Evansville by *30 points.*

A three-game winning streak got us back to 25th before we lost again, this time to a St. Francis (Pa.) team that would finish the season with a losing record (13–15). When we were knocked out in the first round of our conference tournament, it ended any chance of getting back to the NCAA tourney. We accepted a spot in the National Invitation Tournament and reached the quarterfinals before losing 76–74 to Villanova. That the Wildcats went on to win the tournament took a little bit of the sting out of the loss, but I figured that was it for playing basketball;

I couldn't imagine any pro team being interested in someone who couldn't get his team among the 64 invited to the NCAA tourney. Losing in the quarterfinals of the NIT just sealed the thought in my mind that there were plenty of players out there better than me. Time now to see what kind of job I could land with my Xavier degree in organizational communications and whatever having been a local basketball star was worth.

As for Erik Edwards, his career didn't turn out quite the way he hoped. He also stayed at Xavier for four years, but he didn't make it into our regular rotation until his senior year; he went over to play professionally in Europe for a while after graduation. I don't have any ill feelings toward him. I was the underdog. I wasn't supposed to be shit. If anything, I appreciate him for helping push me to show what I could do. He was one of many.

I started preparing my résumé to send to the biggest corporations based in Cincinnati—Procter & Gamble, General Electric, and the Grippo Potato Chip Company—picturing myself in a suit and tie doing the nine-to-five. (Grippo was on the list mainly because their barbecue-flavored chip was, and is, my favorite snack of all time and I imagined bringing bags of it home with me every day. That was my idea of livin' large at the time.)

But the résumés never got sent. Despite not making it to the tournament, several NBA-certified agents called and expressed their interest in representing me. The late Ron Grinker, a Cincinnati-based agent, was the first one to contact me. We met at his office. He told me I might have the potential to be a second-round pick in the NBA draft but more than likely I'd have to pursue a career overseas. Bill Duffy, who is based in Northern California, flew into Cincinnati to meet with me in Coach Gillen's office and had pretty much the same view of my prospects. Both Ron and Bill, independently, suggested that I skip the pre-draft workouts, for fear that they might expose my limitations. They believed tape of what I did in college would be my biggest selling card.

Mark Bartelstein, the third and last agent to call, also flew in to meet with me. He started out by asking what the other agents had said. I told him that they both thought I should skip the pre-draft camp and do a limited number of workouts. "I've watched a lot of tape on you," he said. "I think you're way better than that. You play hard and you've got a nice jumper. You need to work on a few things, but you're not afraid to go get it. I think you could be the surprise of the draft."

I don't know how other players choose an agent, but for me it was pretty simple: Mark believed in me more than anybody else. Including myself.

He also had a radically different view of what I needed to do to convince an NBA team they needed me on their roster. The league's pre-draft combine in Chicago is now the lone pre-draft event where draft prospects gather together for NBA team executives to weigh, measure, interview, and watch play against other draft prospects. Back then, though, the combine was the last of three major events spread across the country— the Portsmouth Invitational in Portsmouth, Virginia; the Desert Classic in Phoenix, Arizona; and the Chicago-based Combine.

Portsmouth is open to anyone who played collegiate basketball, a free-for-all that Mark suggested I skip. Basketball being a team game, there was a chance I could get on a bad team and get dragged down with it. But that also meant Mark had to pull some strings to get me into the Desert Classic, because it was by invitation only and unknowns like myself usually had to prove themselves at Portsmouth to get one.

Mark pulled all sorts of strings to get me in, but that didn't prevent me from nearly walking out halfway through the very first practice session.

The first shock was just how many players were there. Our hotel lobby was packed with dudes from all over the country, a lot of whom I recognized on sight because I'd seen them on TV; they were damn near celebrities to me. Charlie Ward, a two-sport athlete at Florida State, was there despite having won the Heisman Trophy and a national championship as the Seminoles' quarterback. So was Khalid Reeves, a point guard who had just led the University of Arizona to the Final Four. Along with about 70 or so more guys. And me.

A bunch of us were standing in a circle talking, when Stevin Smith, a guard from nearby Arizona State, turned to me and asked how many cards I'd had slipped under my door. It was a pretty basic process—if a team was interested in you, they slipped a card under your hotel door with their logo on it and a note saying they'd like to meet you in Room 826 at a certain time, where they'd put you through the Rorschach ink-blot test and interview you. I was excited that I'd received one from the New York Knicks.

Stevin's nickname was "Hedake," the same way you'd pronounce "headache," and I immediately understood why. "Oh, the Knicks give one to everybody," he scoffed. I didn't say a word, but those feelings of being out of my league came bubbling up in my gut all over again.

I then proved that entering a pre-draft meat market with a shaken confidence is not the ideal approach. The initial workouts were on the Phoenix Suns' practice court, which is tucked in the backside of their arena, a floor below the actual game court. It's like practicing in a cramped basement; the space is not much bigger than the actual court. It felt even more cramped for the workouts because there were chairs lined up side by side all the way around the court and every seat was filled by a scout or GM or coach. More of them sat elbow to elbow in the bleachers section looking down on the court behind one basket. Not the kind of atmosphere recommended for the claustrophobic—or anyone nervous about performing. They split us up into groups of seven to go through some basic drills, with every eye watching our every move.

One shot I never developed that most power forwards and centers have in their repertoire was a jump hook. Of course, that's the first shot they had us shoot, one at a time. I was already fighting my nerves, so when I took that first shot the ball nearly hit the top of the backboard and fell straight down.

It was so unexpected and so far off target that everybody instinctively laughed. I mean everybody—the GMs, the scouts, the other players. Or at least it felt that way. For the rest of the workout, if one GM turned to another to talk, I just assumed it was about me, especially if it looked as if they were amused. After a few minutes, I couldn't take any more of it. I headed for the stairs, fully intending to walk out, fire Mark, and see if I could still land an interview with P&G or Grippo. For whatever reason, one of the other players recognized what I was doing and pulled me back in line for the next drill. Shout out to whoever that was for saving me from my own insecurity.

The rest of the workout, though, didn't go much better. They had us shoot jump shots, starting from around the free-throw line but gradually pushing us farther and farther away from the basket to test our range. I went along with it, but none of this played to my strengths.

After the workout, I called Mark, my eyes watery, and told him what happened. Just as I had to Sister Rose Anne, I told Mark I didn't think I belonged there. He was straightforward with me. "Don't worry about it, Brian, they're not going to draft you or not draft you because of your jump hook. And if you leave now, it will be the biggest mistake of your life. Just show them what you do best and you'll be fine."

The workout was in the morning. That evening we had our first game. K.C. Jones, the late legendary former Boston Celtics' point guard and coach, was in charge of my team. I also had two fast, future NBA point guards, Khalid Reeves and Anthony Goldwire, as teammates. I went to them before we tipped off and asked, "Hey, if I get the damn rebound, hit you with an outlet pass and beat everybody down to the other end, will you give it back?" They looked at each other and exchanged an "is-this-dude-for-real?" look before turning back to me with identical skeptical expressions.

"You're going to get the rebound and then beat everybody down to the other end?"

"That's right," I said. "I'm going to beat everybody."

Reeves shrugged. "If you do that and make it, I'll give it to you all night," he said.

"Bet," I said.

I don't remember the exact figures, but I know I broke 20 in both points and rebounds. And when I got back to the hotel and opened my door, I found a card from every single team lying on the floor. I don't know how many cards Hedake received, I just know he went undrafted. (Ed. note: *Smith's draft status may have been impacted by suspicions he had shaved points as a Sun Devil, which he confessed to doing to the FBI a few years later.*)

My first game was no fluke; I came close to matching that production in the next game. The third team we played finally slowed me down, holding me to 13 points and 16 rebounds. Eric Piatkowski, another small-town Ohio boy (Steubenville) and a sharp-shooting 6'7" wing from the University of Nebraska, won tournament MVP but I made the five-man all-tournament team. I was shocked at how easy it all came to me. It wasn't like the other players weren't working hard; I just knew if I went all-out they couldn't keep up with me chasing rebounds or running down the court—and once I got a sense of that there was no stopping me.

Bartelstein told me my performance in Phoenix had moved me from a possible second-round pick to the top of the second round and possibly even a late first-round pick. But he wasn't ready to settle for that, so if a team called asking me to work out privately for them he agreed to it. Most agents can get a read from talking to GMs what part of the draft their client can expect to be picked and schedule workouts with teams in that range or higher. Mark, though, was committed to moving me up the draft board with every workout. There were 27 teams in the league at the time and I gave a private performance for 15 of them. That's a lot, especially since on some days I worked out for more than one team, or I worked out three days in a row, traveling from city to city in between.

My visit to Philadelphia and a talk with 76ers coach John Lucas is when I first started to believe I had a solid shot at being drafted in the first round. The 76ers had two first-round picks, the sixth and the 20th; I assumed I was there to show I deserved to be the 20th pick. But Mark thought otherwise. "We want to make sure we keep doing these visits," he said. "We've got teams in the lottery talking about you."

Most private workouts consist of going through the kind of drills we did at the Desert Classic and then playing one-on-one or two-on-two with a young assistant coach or other draft prospects. I don't remember who I played one-on-one against in Philly but he was also a big-man draft prospect and I worked that cat.

Afterward, Lucas came up to me and said, "BG, I got to tell you, everything inside me says pick you, but this is my first year and if I do that, they'll crucify me here in Philly."

I understood. The 1994 draft had players like North Carolina center Eric Montross, who a year earlier had won an NCAA championship; local favorite Eddie Jones, a star at Temple; my buddy Khalid Reeves from Arizona; and Jalen Rose, part of

Michigan's Fab Five. A rebounder no one had heard of from an NIT team didn't quite stack up.

"I get it, I get it," I said.

"Man, but you're going to be alright," he said. "Somebody's going to snag you in these top 10 or 15. I wish we could do it."

Lucas probably did more to break down my defenses than anybody. I refused to believe that if he could he'd make me the sixth pick of the entire draft. But I knew I'd had a good workout, and in the place inside where I'd kept myself mentally prepared to go undrafted and head back to Cincinnati looking for a regular job, now I let myself believe someone in the NBA would pick me.

Lakers legend Jerry West, of all people, nearly killed that belief all by himself.

Well, me and a 48-ounce steak might've helped.

"Lottery teams" in the NBA are those that fail to make the playoffs in a given year. Going into the 1994 draft, there were 27 teams in the league; 16 make the playoffs, which means the last 11 are part of a random drawing, or lottery, to determine the draft order.

Even though you're more than likely being picked by a losing team, it's a special distinction as a player to be viewed as a lottery pick. Four West Coast teams had lottery picks in the '94 draft—the Los Angeles Clippers, Los Angeles Lakers, Seattle

SuperSonics, and Sacramento Kings. I worked out for three of them—the Sonics, Kings and Lakers.

The Sonics had a lottery pick despite being anything but a losing team. They had the best regular-season record in the entire league before being upset by the Denver Nuggets in the first round of the playoffs. They owned the rights to the Charlotte Hornets' 1994 first-round pick, however, from a previous trade, and that pick wound up being the 11th and last lottery pick.

George Karl, the head coach, was a former player who never quite shed his playing mindset. He liked to challenge players as if he was still one. My draft workout for him was easily the hardest of any I did. He had me running wind sprints in between drills and every now and then liked to hit you with his shoulder or give you a shove and say, "You ran those pretty good, but are you tough? You a tough guy?" He had this weird smile on his face and then he answered his own question: "Yeah, you're a tough guy." It was a bit overboard, to be honest.

I flew from Seattle down to Sacramento to work out for the Kings. Garry St. Jean was the head coach there but he had the power of a general manager as well. They knew I had a workout for the Lakers the next day in L.A., but before they drove me to the airport we went to dinner at a steakhouse, Morton's. As we looked over the menu to order, St. Jean dared me to eat their 48-ounce steak, which is free if you can finish it. I've never been able to turn down a dare—and I saved the Kings from having to pay for my steak.

But it cost me, big time, the next morning. After dinner, I hopped on a plane to Los Angeles, arriving there sometime around 10:00 PM. My head hit the pillow as soon as I reached my hotel.

I was awakened at 6:00 AM by Lakers assistant coach Michael Cooper banging on my door. I answered it in my underwear, my stomach still trying to digest 48 ounces of meat. "Can I go to the bathroom first?" I asked.

"No!" Cooper said. "This is the Lakers! Let's go!"

The Lakers had their offices at the Great Western Forum, where they played their games, but they used the gym at Loyola Marymount University for practices. That's where Cooper drove me for the workout. I don't remember who they had me work out against, but it was a big 7-foot White kid. He wasn't all that good, but with my entire midsection feeling like concrete, I couldn't move. After about 15 minutes, West, the Lakers general manager at that time, stopped the workout. "For God's sake, stop," he shouted. "What the fuck is wrong with you?" he asked. "Do you not want to play for the Lakers? What is going on?"

I couldn't bring myself to tell him I'd eaten too much steak the night before. It just sounded so lame and unprofessional. So instead, I just shook my head and said, "Nothing."

West was from a small town—Chelyan, West Virginia—just like myself, who had risen to be both one of the greatest guards and general managers of all time. As the model, supposedly, for the NBA logo, he literally had his mark on every ball, backboard, and piece of merchandise. His humble roots and a rough home life had driven him never to be outworked and to constantly strive to identify his weaknesses and fix them. Under different circumstances, we might've had a lot of common experiences to share with each other.

Instead, he was completely disgusted with me and making no bones about it.

"Take him down to the Forum," West said to Cooper.

West, assistant GM Mitch Kupchak, and Lakers legend Magic Johnson met us there. This apparently was where they conducted their pre-draft interviews. Only in my case, they weren't interested in getting to know me as much as they wanted to know what was wrong with me. My sluggish workout did not match what they'd seen from me in college or at the Desert Classic. Maybe they thought I was a victim of the L.A. night life. I didn't want to make excuses, so I didn't say anything.

They sat me in a chair and took turns going in on me for wasting their time. "Who the fuck do you think you are?" one of them asked. "You see them banners out there? You going to come and give that kind of effort?"

"I heard you were good—that ain't good," West sputtered. "That ain't good, son." At one point, he picked up the phone and called St. Jean to ask how my workout went for him.

After he hung up, West seemed to be even more mad. "They said you had a great workout!" he shouted. He was taking it personally that I seemed to be more interested in playing for the Sacramento Kings than the Los Angeles Lakers. "They love you and are ready to take you. But if I have anything to do with it, you'll never play in this league after the shit you pulled on us today!"

I sat there, tears in my eyes, clenching my fists, in part because my stomach was still giving me fits and in part because Jerry freakin' West was vowing to end my NBA career before it ever started. And I had little doubt he had the power to do it.

chapter 4

Everything but the Girl

The 1994 draft was held in Indianapolis, a 2½-hour drive from Cincinnati. The day before the draft, my agent, Mark Bartelstein, called to tell me he had a couple of plane tickets for me.

"First of all, I don't need a plane ticket to get to Indianapolis from Cincinnati," I said. "Second, I'm not going."

Mark was both shocked and disappointed. "Dude, you're going to be top 20, maybe even top 15," he said.

Even though I was confident an NBA team would take me with their first-round pick, I still wasn't sure who; Mark wasn't, either. There is an area at every NBA draft where players, select friends and family members, and their agents sit and wait for their name to be called. They call it "the green room," the same name they use for the waiting room for TV show guests, but at the draft it's not a room but an area just off to the right of the stage with a bunch of tables. The fans in the stands and the TV cameras have full view of everyone as they sit and wait for the commissioner to walk up to the podium and announce their name. A player has to be invited to sit in the green room and the league canvasses the teams to find out who they can feel safe inviting; the last thing anyone wants is to have players and their loved ones squirming in front of an audience as their hopes and dreams slowly evaporate.

I had two fears, then, about the draft—everyone would see me on TV sitting in the green room while one team after another refused to pick me, or I'd get selected and would have to go up on the stage and speak. There was only one way I could make sure none of that happened, and that was by refusing the invitation to attend.

Instead, I had a party in the lobby of a downtown Cincinnati highrise where I was sharing an apartment with Tyrice. We set up two big-screen TVs and invited close to 300 people—family, friends, and former teammates. The draft started and I was talking with everybody, only paying half attention to who was being picked, figuring it would be more than an hour before I heard my name. Then my phone rang. I looked up and the Minnesota Timberwolves had just selected Donyell Marshall from Connecticut with the No. 4 pick. Next up: the Washington Bullets.

I got up and walked to the back of the lobby before I answered. "Hello?"

A voice said: "You ready to be a King?"

"Who is this?"

"Travis Stanley."

"What up, Trav!" Travis was the Kings public relations director.

"We're taking you at eight," he said.

"You're lying."

Travis chuckled. "We're taking you at eight. Is your family near you?"

"No. Not right now."

"Well, don't tell them. Let it be a surprise."

So I hung up and walked back into the party. Everybody stared at me. "We're going 15!" I said. I don't even know if they heard the number—as soon as I said, "We're going," everybody started running up to me and screaming, "Oh my God! I can't believe you really made it to the NBA!"

I remember looking over at my mom and seeing her say, "That's my baby!" My dad sat back and said, "Well, alright." My Uncle John had the biggest reaction.

"I told you!" he shouted. "Remember when I had him out there doing calisthenics and they laughed at him? He's in the fuckin' league now! I told you! Didn't I tell you?"

The only person not jumping up and down was Jermaine. He was looking at me in a funny way because he suspected something was up. He knew teams generally don't call players that far in advance to tell them they were getting picked. The fact that I said I was getting picked 15 and not that I was getting picked by the Indiana Pacers, who owned the 15th pick, also made him understandably suspicious. He just sat there, watching me.

When it came time for the seventh pick by the Clippers, I asked everybody to quiet down. I made the excuse that I wanted to hear if one of my buddies got picked next. For the most part, everybody kept carrying on, except for my mom, dad, and Uncle John, who were sitting next to me on the couch.

About 30 seconds after commissioner David Stern announced that the Clippers had selected Cal's Lamond Murray with the seventh pick and the Sacramento Kings were on the clock, Stern returned to the podium.

"Wait, wait! Listen up!" I told everybody.

"And with the eighth pick in the 1994 NBA draft, the Sacramento Kings select Brian Grant from Xavier University!" Stern announced.

My mom fainted. My uncle sounded as if he was having some kind of spiritual experience, groaning, "Ahhhh!" My grandmother leaned over to slap my mom and wake her up, joyously yelling at her, "Gigi! Get up, Gigi!" I was instantly glad I had decided not to go to Indianapolis. Sure, I missed walking up on the stage and shaking the commissioner's hand and putting on a Sacramento Kings hat and smiling into the cameras, but I wouldn't trade that for being there to see my mom faint and my uncle lose his mind and my dad's proud smile. I still get goosebumps thinking about it.

After they announced I wasn't in attendance, they showed some highlight clips of me playing at Xavier. I sat there and thought about all the twists and turns that led to this day— Mr. Martt's second chance, the anonymous caller to Xavier, Mo Brantley missing a class, Mark believing in me (and me believing Mark), not walking out of that Desert Classic workout, even the 48-ounce steak—and I started to choke up, realizing how lucky I truly was.

Less than 24 hours later, I found out the Kings' fans weren't feeling quite as lucky. In a way, I wasn't, either.

The Kings sent a convertible limousine to the airport to take me to the arena for an introductory press conference. Our driver had the radio tuned to the local AM sports radio station and the team's flagship, KHTK. I don't know who the Kings' fans were hoping their team would draft—maybe Michigan's Jalen Rose or North Carolina's Eric Montross—but it certainly wasn't "a little known power forward from Xavier," which is how a lot of the mock drafts described me. One caller after another ripped the Kings—GM Geoff Petrie in particular—for picking me.

To be fair to the fans, this was the Kings' sixth year in a row with a lottery pick. The first was in 1989, when they took center Pervis "Never Nervous" Ellison with the No. 1 pick. He lasted one season and had his nickname changed to "Out of Service" after injuries limited him to 34 games before the Kings shipped him to Washington in a three-team deal that netted a future first-round pick from the Utah Jazz, a couple of veteran players (Bobby Hansen and Erick Leckner) and a couple of future second-round picks. Quite the haul, but none of the new pieces amounted to anything significant in a Kings' uniform.

They had four first-round picks the next season, led by No. 7 Lionel Simmons, their starting small forward the next four years but never an All-Star. They did better the next season by trading the third overall pick, Syracuse's Billy Owens, on draft night, to the Golden State Warriors for future six-time All-Star shooting guard Mitch Richmond. But then they took another small forward with the seventh pick in 1992, grabbing Walt Williams over future seven-time champion Robert Horry and All-Star guard Latrell Sprewell. They picked seventh again in '93, taking Duke point guard Bobby Hurley, who had a legendary career for the Blue Devils but struggled as a pro before a car accident halfway through his rookie year ended it and nearly killed him. He made it back to play 3½ more seasons before being dealt to, and eventually waived by, the Vancouver Grizzlies. After starting all 19 games before the accident he spent the rest of his career as a back-up.

I didn't care if the Kings' history justified them hating me or not. Once again, I faced an army of doubters. I can still hear those callers verbally smacking me in the face right along with the California spring air as we cruised down the highway to Arco Arena.

"We did it again," one caller said. "What the hell was Geoff thinking?"

And another: "We wasted an eighth pick on some unknown from Xavier?"

Tyrice, who I invited to come along, looked at me, cocking his head and raising his eyebrows. The driver went to turn off the radio, but I stopped him.

"It's alright, keep it on," I said. "I want to hear this." What the driver didn't know is that the callers were filling my tank, the same way the people in Georgetown did. And the North-South organizers. And Erik Edwards. And Hedake.

If the fans weren't sure about me on draft night, though, they got even saltier as contract negotiations dragged on through the summer and into training camp. The assumption was that I wanted more money than the Kings were offering, but that wasn't it. I've never told anyone (other than my agent) the real reason until now.

It had to do with a girl. Kelly, my college girlfriend.

The day after I was drafted, she called me.

"You know, I'm so happy for you, Brian," she said.

"Thank you, Kelly. Where you at?"

"I'm at home." She paused. "Listen, I just want to tell you that I know you were never loyal to me the whole time we were together. I know you were cheating on me and I can't expect that you'll never not cheat on me. So don't ever call me again." Click. That was it. The day after the happiest day of my life, my girlfriend broke up with me. Over the phone. This was opposite of how I thought it was supposed to go; I thought once you got drafted in the NBA you were supposed to get girls, not lose them.

Did I mess around on Kelly? Sure did. I'm not proud of it, but I showed up at Xavier not really knowing what an honest, healthy relationship between a boy and girl looked like. Growing up in Georgetown, sneaking around and dating on the sly was how it was done. There weren't a lot of available girls, so when you were lucky enough to hook up with one, you had the eagle eye on her to make sure she didn't step out on you. And if you could mess around with more than one? There was no shame in that; with the pickings so slim, it was actually something you could brag about. At least that's how me and my cousins saw it.

Kelly knew I was messing around while we were dating—and I know she knew. So I figured on some level she was alright with it. I can look back now and see how immature I was, how someone tolerating something doesn't make it right, but at the time I was just a young dude who not only suddenly found girls interested in him but could freely show his interest in them whenever he wanted. I went from having a hard time getting any girl to talk to me to having some of the prettiest chasing me. It was as if I were a kid with his nose pressed up against the ice cream store window for years without a dime in his pocket and then suddenly the manager had invited me in and offered samples of whatever I wanted.

I left Kelly alone for about two weeks. I told myself I didn't care, there were other fish in the sea, and my new wealth and fame were giving me one big damn net. Mark flew out to Sacramento and helped me and Jermaine find a place to live—a duplex—and set me up with a car dealership, which loaned me a two-door Yukon. We drove it back to a completely empty duplex, suddenly realizing we had no food or furniture. All I had brought with me was as many clothes as I could fit into a big bag. We roughed it, sleeping on the floor that night. The next day we connected with Kings' guard LeBradford Smith, who lived down the street with his wife. (Ed. note: *LeBradford's claim to fame from his three NBA seasons is scoring 37 points against Michael Jordan and the Chicago Bulls in a rare back-to-back home-and-home two-game regular-season series. A revenge-seeking Jordan scored 36 the next night—in the first half—on his way to 47 points while holding LeBradford to 15.*)

LeBradford's wife made dinner for us and lent us pillows, blankets, a TV, and a DVD player. A few days later I went shopping for a couple of beds and a few pieces of furniture. What more does a bachelor crib need?

LeBradford also clued me in on the best summer run in Sacramento for pick-up basketball. It was in a Salvation Army gym not far from where we lived. Kings' players would drop in for some five-on-five action with the local legends and a few ex-college players. I got the same treatment from them the first time I walked into the gym that I did from the KHTK callers. "There goes that bum they drafted," I overheard someone say.

Duane Causwell, a 7-foot, 240-pound center and the third of the Kings' four first-round picks in 1990, was on the other team in my first run. He wasn't the one who called me a bum but it didn't matter—the first time I got the ball I dunked on him. I threw a few more down on him before the game was over.

"Damn, you didn't have to get on me like that," he complained afterward.

I didn't say anything, but in my head I thought: *Yeah, I did.*

The routine became: get an afternoon run in at the Salvation Army, invite everyone over to the duplex for a barbecue afterward, listen to music and hang until everybody went home, pop a movie into the DVD player, crash—and then do it all over again. One day, a regular at the pick-up games, Chuck Terrell, pulled me aside during one of the post-run get-togethers and said, "Brian, you've got to stop inviting all these cats over."

"Why? What do you mean?"

"Some of them are Crips. And some of them are Bloods. If you're not careful, you're going to have a gang war jump off in your living room."

I looked around and suddenly sensed a tension I hadn't been aware of before. That wasn't something we ever had to worry about at the Dust Bowl in Maysville or at the Ripley courts. We knew about the Bloods and the Crips, but there weren't any gangs or turf wars at that time anywhere in southern Ohio. Hoopin' and having a barbecue for everyone afterward was just something you did.

I saw some cats looking around my place in a way I hadn't noticed before, either, as if they were casing it. It probably helped that the place looked like it had been decorated by a couple of guys who didn't know anything about interior decorating. I kept going to the Salvation Army runs but took Chuck's advice and put an end to the open-invitation barbecues. I was nervous for a couple of weeks that some of the fellas might invite themselves over while we weren't home, if you know what I mean, but nothing ever happened.

If you're in the NBA or basketball circles, you've probably heard of Chuck—he was a longtime marketing representative for Nike and a close confidant of NBA stars Kevin Durant and Kyrie Irving. He was just starting out when we met in Sacramento, but I think he recognized that Jermaine and me were small-town guys and looked out for us. I was lucky to meet him when I did.

I sometimes wonder what would have happened if I had been drafted by one of the teams in L.A., New York, or Miami. It was pretty easy to get over on me in those days. I was at a gas station, filling up the Yukon, when a guy pulled up and offered to sell me a new laptop computer, dirt cheap. It was still in the box, all nice and neat. I figured he'd stolen it, but I didn't ask any questions. I drove home, opened the box and found a brick neatly wrapped inside.

Despite the routine and meeting plenty of people, I couldn't stop thinking about Kelly. I reached her on the phone once.

"What the hell is wrong with you?" I asked.

"Don't call me again." Click. I didn't listen. Flip phones had just become a thing, so I was mostly calling her home phone. When her parents answered, they'd tell me she didn't want to talk or she wasn't there. They weren't mean or mad, which I appreciated; that they were big Xavier supporters—her dad was a Xavier alum—might've had something to do with that.

Kelly and I first met at the Xavier basketball awards banquet my junior year. They were sitting at the same table with me, my mom, and my grandmother. Kelly and I were seated next to each other. "I see you looking at that girl," my grandmother whispered to me. "You better stop that."

A few months later, Kelly toured the campus and they invited me to join them. After that, Kelly would swing by with some of her high school girlfriends to hang out and listen to music. Covington, Kentucky, which is just on the other side of the Ohio River from Cincinnati, is known for its night clubs and a lot of Black folk are known to hang out in them. Kelly let it be known that she liked hanging out there, too. A signal, of sorts.

"Okay, alright," I said. Signal received.

"You're really nice," she said. "I'm not really dating anybody. I *was* dating this dude named Lee."

"Cool."

She was very pretty, but she was still in high school, so I wasn't about to do anything more than be friendly. I lost track of her over the summer. Then, one day at the start of my senior year I was walking across campus to the cafeteria and I saw this little cutie in cut-off shorts and Birkenstocks with her blond hair pulled back and bushed out in back. "Damn, that's Kelly," I thought to myself. I ended up calling her and we started dating. They had me over to their house all the time for holidays and dinners and took me for who I was, not the color of my skin. I hadn't had too many experiences like that, so it meant a lot.

The summer came and went, the start of the Kings' training camp was fast approaching, and I still hadn't signed a contract. "You need to be there for the start of training camp," Mark said.

Instead, I flew to Cincinnati and went to a Xavier house party where I knew I could run in to Kelly. I was sitting with a couple of my former Xavier teammates when Kelly came strolling into view holding hands with another student I didn't recognize. I was both mad and jealous and jumped into my car and left. I got her on the phone later that night. "I'm not seeing that guy," she said. "But you had your chance and you blew it."

I flew back to Sacramento thinking, *There's a reason she was trying to make me jealous. This isn't over.*

Meanwhile, Mark had convinced the Kings to sweeten their offer. "This is pretty good money," he said. "You need to be at the first preseason game."

But Kelly wasn't an itch I had finished scratching. I flew back to Cincinnati again to give it one more shot. This time she was willing to see me, inviting me over to the house to watch *Friends*, but that was it and I wanted to be more than friends. I finally accepted it was over between us and flew back to Sacramento.

Which was good, because the Kings had given Mark an ultimatum.

"Alright," Mark said. "I got you $29 million over 13 years. The Kings are saying either take it or enjoy your career playing overseas."

"Okay," I said. "I'll take it."

"Thank God," Mark said.

I signed in time to play in the final exhibition game and St. Jean didn't hesitate to throw me out there. The fans, thinking this power forward they'd never heard of had the audacity to hold out for more money when he should be grateful he's in the league at all, booed. Loudly. To make matters worse, flying back and forth between Cincinnati and Sacramento had not left me in very good playing shape. We were playing their biggest rival, the Warriors. Those callers I heard riding in the droptop limo were still on my mind, along with the boo birds. Playing center for the Warriors was 7'7" Manute Bol, who retired with more blocked shots than points scored. The combination of his height and a wingspan of 8'6" made him a challenge to score on around the rim. What better way to shut up everyone than to dunk on the man with the second-best career average for blocked shots (3.3 per game)?

The only problem was, I didn't have enough of my usual spring to get the job done. Three times I tried to dunk on him and all three times he swatted my shot. The cheers from the disgruntled Kings' fans got louder with each one. I made a couple of jump shots, but they didn't care about that. I might be wearing a Kings' uniform, but I was clearly the enemy.

Mark saw me after the game and said, "Man, you've got nerves of steel. You were really holding out for that money."

That's when I realized I had never shared with Mark anything about Kelly. Every time he'd call and lay out the Kings' offer, I'd say, "Nah, that ain't cool. They can do better than that."

So he'd say something to the effect of, "Yeah, you're right. Let me get back to you." But the real reason is I wasn't ready to focus on playing basketball until I got Kelly back—or, as it turned out, knew I couldn't.

"You think I was holding out for more money?"

"Why? If that wasn't it, what was it?"

"My fucking girlfriend broke up with me and I was trying to get her back."

"You fucking—you did *what?* Oh God. Do me a favor. Don't ever tell anybody that."

I eventually got into shape and worked my way into the Kings fans' hearts. Although it's the state capitol, Sacramento has a small-town vibe and is surrounded by farms and agriculture. They kind of felt like my people.

A few months after Kelly dumped me, the team had me make a community appearance at a local mall. As Jermaine and I descended on an escalator toward the ground floor where an area had been cordoned off for the event, we saw the Kings' dancers lined up. My eyes locked on this one brown-skinned girl. I pointed her out to Jermaine.

"Man, you see that Mexican girl down there?" I asked.

"Oh, yeah."

"Wooo, boy, I'd love to meet a girl like her. I could marry her."

Two things about team dancers you may or may not know: 1) they don't make much money as team dancers—certainly not enough to live off of—so they have other full-time jobs, and

2) they're not allowed to date players on the team. What is the chance that being forced to sneak around would discourage a guy from Georgetown with my history?

I came up with the idea of writing her a letter and having a friend give it to her. But one of the other dancers saw the hand-off going down and heard my name and said, "No, Gina. Don't do it. He's not going to get you fired."

So she didn't accept the letter and I began thinking maybe it just wasn't meant to be. But Gina proved to be more resourceful than I was. A few weeks later, a buddy of mine comes up to me and says, "Hey, man, I've got a message for you."

"Yeah?"

"You know that girl Gina?"

"Yeah."

"Well, she was at an appearance and didn't have a ride home, so I gave her one."

I tilted my head at him as if to say, "Do I really want to hear this?"

He understood what I was thinking. "No, no, it was nothing like that," he said. "She actually leaned over and said, 'Could you give Brian my number?' And I told her, 'Oh, yeah. I'll give it to Brian. He likes you. You know he likes you, right?'"

I'd pointed her out to all the guys on the team, so it wasn't exactly a secret. Anyway, my buddy gave me the number and I finally talked to Gina on the phone. That's how I found out it was her first year dancing and her regular job was working at the Baby Gap in a trendy downtown mall.

When my former Xavier teammate Aaron Williams came into town with the Milwaukee Bucks, I showed him around and suggested we swing by the complex and drop in on a girl I was hoping to date. Seemed like a decent cover in case anyone saw me talking to her.

Gina had her eyes on Aaron from the minute we walked into the store. Walked right up to him and said, "Hi." This was the first time Gina and I were face to face, only it seemed she was more interested in Aaron's face. They chit-chatted and I finally said, "Alright, we're going."

She said, "Okay," without even looking at me.

After we left, Aaron said, "You mind if I get at her?"

I was pissed. At her, not him. "Nah, dude. Do whatever you want."

I enjoy pain, so I even decided to be the facilitator. When I finally talked to Gina, I said, "Let me give you my boy Aaron's number."

"What? What do you mean?"

"Well, you were all in his fucking face."

"Oh my God. No. I couldn't look at you. I was too scared, so I kept looking at him."

"Well, he's asking for your number. I could just give you his."

"No, don't. You. You're the one."

That's how it started and that's how it was for the better part of our relationship. We fell hard for each other. When I told her later about what I told Jermaine on the escalator when I laid eyes on her for the first time, she said she said something similar to her cousin the first time she saw me.

She was living in Livermore at the time, but she'd already made the dance team and was watching my introductory press conference as she packed to move to Sacramento. She'd also already been told the dance team rules and regulations, including the one forbidding a relationship with any of the players.

"Oh, my God," she said. "Come here, Danielle. Look at the new rookie."

Her cousin didn't have quite the same reaction. "Oh, okay," she said.

But Gina didn't care. "Call me fired," she told her cousin. "If I see him, it's on."

And so it was. It was on. And off. And on again. We were hot for each other and sometimes we were just hot. We loved each other so much, sometimes we hated each other.

This is a scene that played out many times almost from the start. Details might change—why we were fighting, what we said or did to piss off each other—but the chain of events were basically the same. She'd be mad at me about something—probably deservedly so—and stomp out of my apartment to her car with me right behind her.

"I hate you!" she'd yell as she climbed into her car.

I'd throw something at her car—one time it was a bag of gym shoes at her windshield—and yell, "Forget you!"

"Oh, that's real mature," she'd say. "Shut up. We're done." And then she'd speed off.

By 10:00 or 11:00 that night, one of us would be calling the other and saying, "I'm sorry," and the other would say, "I'm sorry, too," and then it would be either, "Want to come back over?" or, "Can I come back over?" and the answer would always be yes.

There were a lot more fun times than rough ones. Jermaine was living with me and although Chuck had a house in Stockton with his mother, he was always hanging out at my place. Another cousin from Georgetown, Mike Gallagher, came out and lived at my place for a while, too.

It eventually came time to choose. All my guys liked Gina, but she got on their nerves, too. She liked to talk shit. We'd all get ready to go out to dinner or to a club and Gina would say to Chuck or Jermaine or Mike, "You're wearing that?"

Finally, one of them said, "Hey, brother, when is she leaving?"

"I don't know, man. I kind of like having her over."

They rolled with it for a while, but then the complaints ramped up.

"I can't stand this chick," one of them said. "She's always jumping on my back."

So I came up with a plan. I drove them by Gina's apartment near the arena. "She's going to move her stuff in with me and you guys move over here," I said.

That clearly shocked them. "We've got to move out of the house?"

"I just think it would be best. Y'all will have your own space and you don't even have to pay rent. I got it."

But they understood. I'd made my choice. They were just like, "Yeah, whatever, man."

Nothing really changed. Gina and I both enjoyed when it was just the two of us, but we didn't get much alone time. Mike, Jermaine, and Chuck still hung out at my place all the time, especially after the Kings drafted Corliss Williamson the next year and Corliss moved in across the street. He had a pool table at his place, so they were either at his place or mine. I was the same—when I needed to get out of the house, I'd walk across the street, shoot some pool, watch TV, have a beer, and then walk back home.

There was one problem with my duplex—it was haunted. My mom came out on a visit and one afternoon asked, "Why did you tell me to go get in bed?"

It seemed like an odd question. "When?"

"Last night."

"I never came downstairs."

She had fallen asleep on the couch. After waking up, she heard someone walk up behind her and say, "Go lay in your bed upstairs." She said she sat there for a minute and then got up and looked around because she never heard anyone go back up the stairs.

I asked the woman who lived on the other side of our duplex if she had experienced anything weird happening where she lived.

"No," she said, "but I think the people who lived there before you talked about some weird stuff happening."

"Well, I think we need to have this place blessed."

My neighbor was cool with that idea and invited her pastor over to do the job and we didn't have any problems with ghosts after that. But we still had problems. My jealousy caused a lot of them.

Since we couldn't risk anyone finding out we were dating and Sacramento had a relatively limited social scene back then, we'd either stay in at my place or make the two-hour drive down to San Francisco. Gina was the first to take me to the famous Pier 39 and its stinky sea lions. We did all the touristy things, like ride a trolley car and jump in the instant photo booth. I was 22 and she was 19. Young, dumb love at its finest. In some ways, I was more young-minded than her. I wasn't the best-looking kid growing up. It started with my long arms, long legs, and

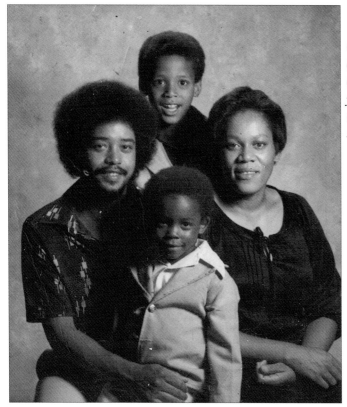

Grant family portrait (1979): my dad, Thomas (left); me (top); my younger brother, Brandon (bottom); and my mom, Dorella (right).

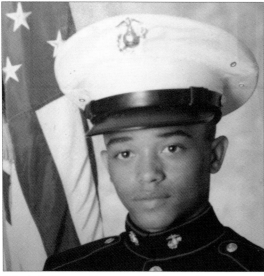

My dad, Thomas Grant, in his Marine Corps picture (1973).

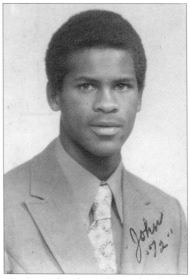

Here's Uncle John (John Richard Bennett) in his 1972 high school senior photo.

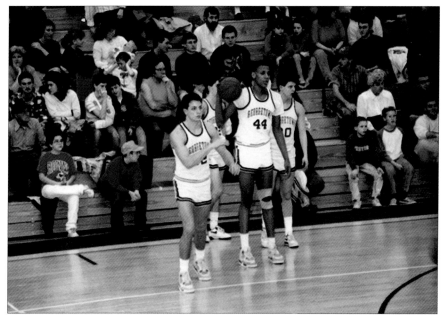

Here I am (middle) with a couple teammates—Eddie Johnson (left) and Jamie Johnson (right)—in a 1989 high school game.

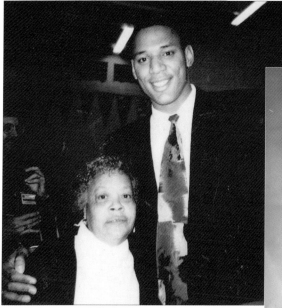

Me and Mamaw (Gladys) Grant at a college banquet in 1993.

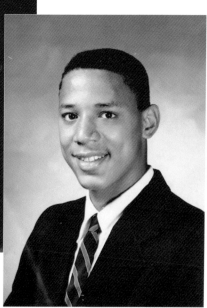

My high school graduation picture (1990).

Me at my college graduation in 1994, receiving my diploma from the president of Xavier University.

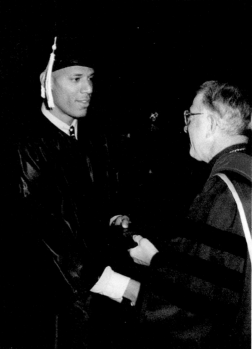

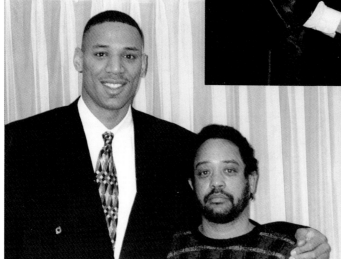

Me and my dad at my college graduation.

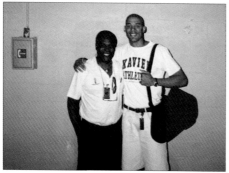

Here I am at the Desert Classic pre-NBA Draft camp in 1994, with my coach at the Classic, K.C. Jones.

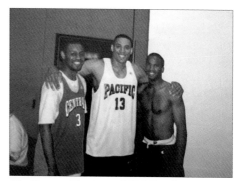

The Dessert Classic pre-NBA Draft camp in 1994, with camp teammates Adrian Autry (left) and Khalid Reeves (right).

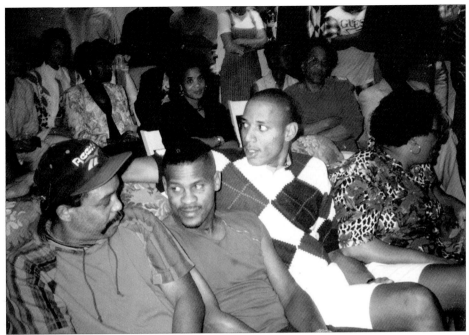

Family and friends at my 1994 NBA Draft party in Cincinnati.

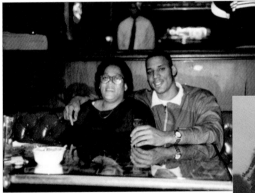

Dinner with my favorite woman in the world, my mom (1995).

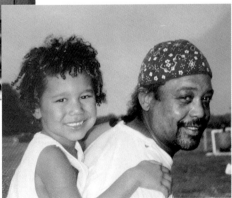

Summertime in Ohio: my dad with his grandson Elijah.

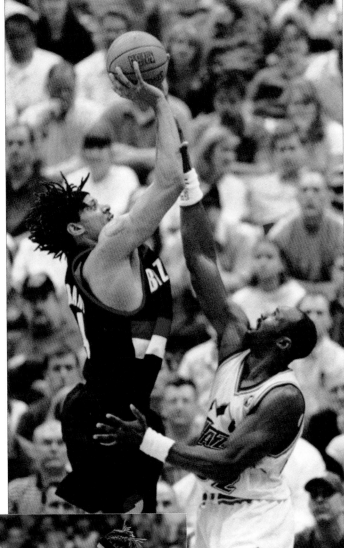

Me shooting over Karl Malone in one of our many battles.
(AP Images/Jack Smith)

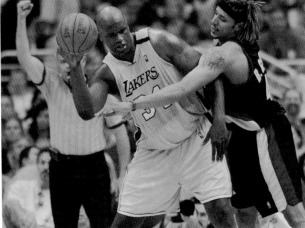

Going toe-to-toe with Shaq in Game 1 of the 2000 Western Conference finals.
(AP Images/Mark J. Terrill)

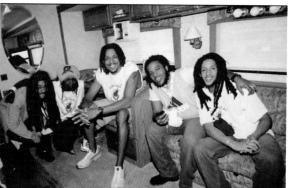

With the Marley family and friends at the Miami Heat Family Festival in 2002. From left, Damian Marley, Mr. Cheeks, me, Stephen Marley, and Julian Marley.

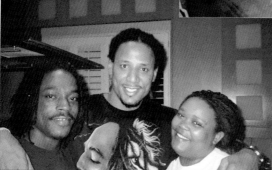

In my Miami home in 2002 with my brother Brandon and my sister Brianna.

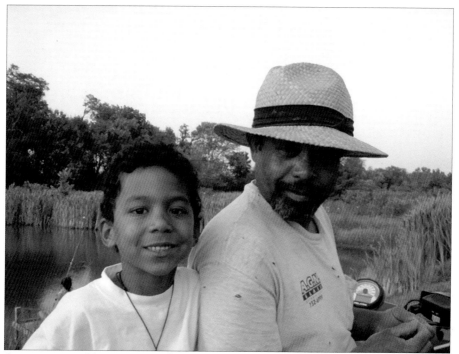

Summertime in Ohio: my son Jaydon with his Papaw Tommy.

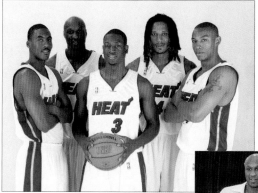

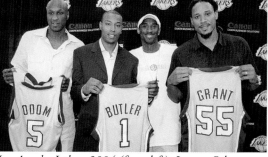

Starting-five photo, Miami Heat media day for the 2003–04 season (from left): Eddie Jones, Lamar Odom, Dwyane Wade, me, and Caron Butler.

Los Angeles Lakers 2004 (from left): Lamar Odom, Caron Butler, Kobe Bryant, and me.

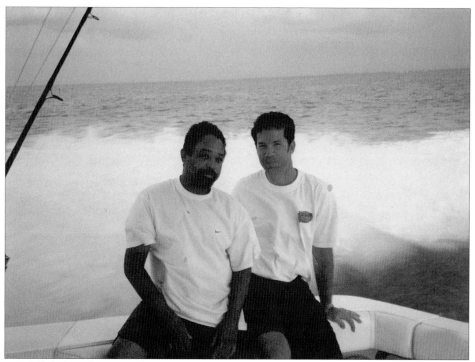

My dad (left) and my great friend and natural healer, Phillipe Manicom (right), on a fishing trip on my boat in 2004.

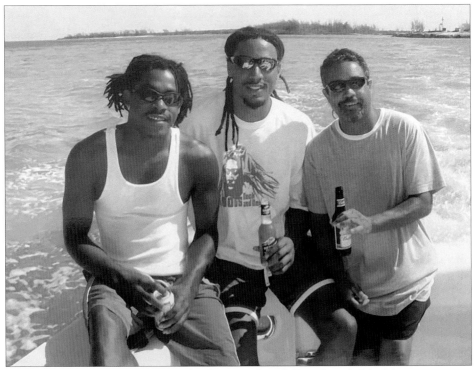

Bahamas Guys Trip (2005), with my brother, Brandon, (left) and my dad (right).

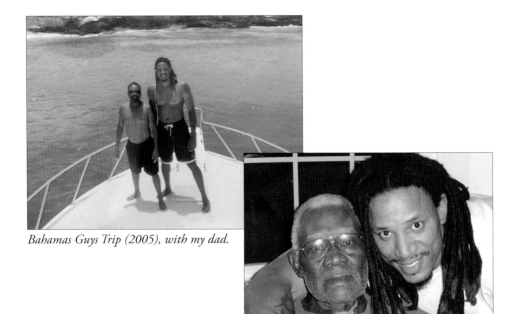

Bahamas Guys Trip (2005), with my dad.

Me and Papaw (Tom) Bennett at a 2006 family reunion.

short torso, all of it accentuated by my growth spurt, which, combined with us being on a very tight budget, resulted in me wearing clothes that didn't fit. I also cut my own hair and tried to give myself the Bobby Brown cut. The front looked dope but anybody who saw me from the back would go, "Yo, the slant ain't slanted!"

All of that made me insecure about my looks and the imprint never quite left me. I had it so bad for Gina that I felt a need to prepare for someone trying to take her from me. I'd make up situations and ask her how she'd react in them. For example, I once created this scenario for her:

"You're going out with your girlfriends. You're at the bar and all of a sudden your ex-boyfriend comes up and says, 'Can I buy you a drink?' What do you say?"

"Yeah," Gina said.

"Wrong answer," I told her. "And I'm going to tell you why. I'm going to put myself in your ex-boyfriend's shoes.

"I see my ex-girlfriend, Gina, and she is looking goooood. Let me go up and say 'hi' to her, offer to buy her a drink and see what's up. 'Hey, Gina, good to see you. What are you drinking? Let me get you one.' She says, 'Sure.' Now I'm thinking, 'She accepted my drink. Cool.'

"Then she starts telling me about how she's in love with Brian Grant, you know, Kings rookie, this, that, and the other. I don't take that as, 'I've moved on and am not interested, thank you.' I take that as a challenge; as in, maybe she's just trying to make me jealous. And I'm thinking, 'I won her once, let's see if I can do it again.' Why else would she accept my drink? So now I'm going to go to work.'"

Gina had this confused, incredulous look on her face. "Is this school?" she asked.

I kept going. "So this is what you might want to watch out for," I said, switching back into the imaginary ex-boyfriend role.

"Oh, I'm so happy for you. You know, when we were together, man, I wish I'd have done the right things, but you're happy and I'm happy for you—let me buy your girls a drink too."

"Now," I said, "your girls might like me or they might not like me, but they're not going to pass up a free drink. So they say to you, 'Yeah, girl, let's have a drink.'

"Now we're all drinking and the girlfriends know I'm available but I'm not acting like it. My attention is on you. And you're thinking, 'That's how it should be.' And then you might think, 'Well, Brian's attention wasn't fully on me the last time we all went out…' And that starts to bring up some old feelings."

I would pose these scenarios all the time. "Who thinks like that?" Gina asked, more than once.

And every time my answer was, "I do."

The first major stress test of her commitment to me came about five months after we started dating and a couple of months into my rookie season. After one of our early games, Jermaine nudged me. "Hey, that girl's looking at you," he said. I looked over at her and smiled. She waved and smiled back.

"I've got to leave," I told Jermaine, "but you can get her number if you want." So he did and then passed it on to me. That's how I met Amanda.

We might never have hooked up if not for the weather. The team was returning from a road trip when fog prevented us from landing in Sacramento. Instead, we landed at the Oakland airport and the team arranged for a bus to drive us home. I still had Amanda's number on me and I knew she lived in Oakland. She said she was close by. I asked if anybody on the team wanted to go with me. Walt Williams took me up on the offer. Amanda showed up with a 12-pack of beer, drove us to Sacramento, dropped off Walt, and then drove to my duplex. I knew Gina was out of town with a girlfriend. I invited Amanda to come in for a minute.

We had put a hot tub out on the duplex deck and Jermaine and Chuck were hanging out in it when I walked in with Amanda. Jermaine, in particular, didn't like what was happening. As soon as he could get a minute with me alone he said, "What did you bring her here for?"

"Our plane got re-routed to Oakland. I was stranded. She gave me a ride home."

"C'mon, man, you know what I'm sayin'. I mean, you can do what you want, but Gina better not find out about her coming here. This is home, man."

When Amanda left, she asked, "You're not going to call me, are you?"

"I'll call you," I said.

I didn't talk to Amanda again until she called me two months later and said she was pregnant and that I was about to be a dad. I called Gina as soon as we hung up. "Listen, this girl just called me and said that she's pregnant and that it's mine," I said. "I don't know if it is or isn't, but if it is my child, you have to know I'm not going to not be with my kid." I might've been short a few morals but I was not going to abandon a child that was mine.

"When was it?" Gina asked. I told her. "We were seeing each other!"

"Yeah, but I don't think we were doing anything."

"Who cares? We were seeing each other!"

"Well, I'm telling you now. This would be a good time to get out of this relationship if that's what you want."

She didn't say anything for a minute. "No, I'm going to stick it out," she said. "She's probably just lying."

I took a DNA test. It came back as a 99.9 percent match. She wasn't lying. Seven months later, my first son, Amani, was born. I had no intention or desire to leave Gina for Amanda, but

I also planned to be as much of a dad to Amani as I could. Gina, God bless her, stuck it out—but she was now on high alert.

Timing, they say, is everything. That goes for bad timing, too. Jermaine's girlfriend from Georgetown came out and visited us. Gina was her usual life-of-the-party, bubbly self. "Oh, my God," Jermaine's girlfriend said. "I like her. She is so beautiful."

A couple days after she flew back to Georgetown, Kelly happened to call Jermaine's girlfriend.

"How's Jermaine?" Kelly asked.

"He's good."

"I don't really need to know how Brian's doing, but how's he doing?"

"He is dating this girl, she is so beautiful. Her name is Gina. I think this might be the one."

Two days later, my phone rings. "Brian, this is Kelly," the voice on the other end says. "Can you talk for a minute?"

Gina was sitting on the bed right next to me. "Uh…" I said. Gina's antennae went up immediately.

"Who is that?"

"Uh, yeah, I can," I said to Kelly.

"Who *is* that?" Gina asked again.

"It's Kelly," I said. I had told Gina all about what had happened right after the draft.

"Hang up the phone right now."

"I'm not hanging up the phone."

"Then I'm gone." She got up and left.

Kelly explained why she refused to get back together with me. "If I hadn't done that, you would've never respected me," she said.

"I know," I said. "But I met somebody."

"I know, but I just want you to know that I talked to my parents and I convinced them to let me come out and stay with you over spring break," she said. This was big for both Kelly and her parents because they were devout Christians and that meant they were trusting me and her to do the right thing.

She didn't stop there. "I just want you to know that I will always love you," she said, "and I want to be with you."

Now it was my turn to tell her she had blown it. "Too late," I said.

"Oh, no."

"You're too late. Sorry."

That was another night where Gina eventually came back. By the end of the season, we didn't want to sneak around anymore. Gina met with the dance team supervisor/coach and said, "I'm going to have to quit the team."

The supervisor said, "I already know."

"Know what?" Gina said.

"You've been seeing Brian Grant all year."

"How'd you know?"

"Never mind how I know. I only recently found out about it. I didn't fire you because you're my best dancer and you helped me choreograph quite a few things. I figured as long as you kept it quiet, then I didn't have to do anything. But you can't come back next year if you're going to continue to see him."

"I understand," Gina said. "I'm done."

I couldn't wait to take Gina everywhere to show her off. First I took her home to Georgetown, just knowing everybody was going to be like, "Damn!" Which is exactly what happened. My family just loved her. Then I took her to Jamaica, where I fell hard for a second time. Only this time it wasn't for a woman.

My family was worried I'd lost my way; I was convinced I'd finally found it.

chapter 5
Rasta Mon

Music has shaped how I see the world and my place in it since I was a kid. Seeing my story in the Pet Shop Boys' "West End Girls" was only one example. When I was growing up, my dad and Uncle Tom Lightfoot used to spin records in this hole-in-the-wall bar in the basement of a house over in Maysville. I'm sure they didn't have a liquor license, but they'd pay the two of them $40 to work as DJs. They'd play Earth, Wind & Fire, the Ohio Players, the Isley Brothers, and Midnight Star. My mom liked light classic rock—Joni Mitchell, the Carpenters, Bread—and would sing along with it around the house. Glam rock was the jam at the high school—Warrant, Mötley Crüe, Guns N' Roses, Whitesnake, Lita Ford. That's what I listened to the most, but I couldn't really connect with it.

When Afrika Bambaataa, a DJ out of the Bronx in New York who's considered the godfather of electrofunk and hip-hop, came out with an underground hit called "Planet Rock," my whole identity as a Black kid surrounded by White people changed. It wasn't confrontational, but it was revolutionary. Then N.W.A. came along and took it another step, giving a voice to being Black and feeling oppressed. The idea stunned us: You mean being treated like shit for being Black isn't just a Georgetown thing? I was 16 years old when N.W.A.'s first album, *Straight Outta Compton*, was released, and I heard some cats all the way out in California expressing all the same thoughts and feelings I had about people automatically labelling me as a bad person simply because I was Black and poor. My cousins and I ran around Georgetown calling each other by the street names of the N.W.A. rappers—Eazy E, Ice Cube, and Ren. I was DJ Yella, or Yellow Boy. For the first time in my life, there was an element to being Black that was cool.

That spark of rebellion might be why I quit the marching band my junior year in high school. I dreamed of being a saxophone player after I heard the saxophone solo in Men at Work's "Who Can It Be Now," but we couldn't afford to buy an instrument so I played the drums with Jermaine. One day we were goofing around in practice, throwing drumsticks at each other, and a stick accidentally clipped a girl clarinetist. The band director pulled us into his office and said that he was going to give us two swats each. I refused to let him.

"Do I have to call your mom?" he asked.

"Go ahead," I said.

He did. After explaining to my mom the situation, he handed me the phone. My mom usually had my back, but she didn't this time. "You can either take the two swats or you will be grounded for two weeks," she said. "And by grounded I mean go to school and come straight home afterward. No use of the car, no going outside after you get home, no seeing your friends."

I consented to the two swats. I swear before he gave me the first one, he went into the other room and got pumped up because it stung so bad I had to walk around for a minute with my eyes watering. It was as if he had been waiting his entire life to give me those licks, because the second one was worse.

"Screw you!" I shouted before I limped out of his office. "I quit!"

Music usually served as a way for me to connect with people I otherwise wouldn't. Developing a taste for hard rock from my White high school friends, soft rock from my mom, R&B from my dad, and then rap and hip-hop with my cousins left me with an open mind when I got to the Xavier campus. I didn't care as much about what kind of music it was as much as how it made me feel and if the song seemed to be about some aspect of my life.

My friendship with Raphael Saadiq resulted in an actual song about my life, though not a part I might've chosen for him to sing about if I'd had a choice.

I met Raphael a few months into my NBA career quite by accident. I was at a stop light with the top down on my convertible coupe when a dude on a bright yellow Harley-Davidson motorcycle pulled up next to me. He recognized me and I asked him if he wanted to grab something to eat at a Mexican joint I liked. It turned out he had a house in Sacramento and had built a recording studio in it.

"How you like it here?" he asked.

"It's alright, once I got used to them booing me," I said.

"They ain't booing you now, though, are they?"

We felt as if we had a lot in common—two young brothers from very humble beginnings who had just hit the big time and weren't exactly sure how to deal with everything coming at us. He was from Oakland, one of 14 kids, and had seen a lot more than any young kid should ever see. I had just made it to the NBA, and along with being in the R&B group Tony! Toni! Toné!, he had dropped a solo hit, "Ask of You." I never knew who I might see at his house when I dropped by—D'Angelo, P Diddy—but it was a thrill to roll in and watch them work together. I guess it would be a bit like someone getting a chance to come in and watch an NBA team practice.

Nothing affected me more, though, than the musical lesson I received on my first trip to Jamaica. I went as a vacation after my rookie year with the Kings. I didn't know anything about the island, other than it was where Bob Marley was from, but I was interested in the food and people and the general vibe. So Gina and I talked to a travel agent and booked an eight-day stay at the Sandals Resort in Ochos Rios.

One night, we left the resort and went out on the town to experience some of the local flavor. I wore a custom linen suit I'd had made just for the trip—a tan sleeveless suit jacket and matching pants, the exact outfit you'd expect some dumb tourist from the States to wear. Gina wore a nice dress. We walked into a hole-in-the-wall bar and ordered drinks. Everyone had on flip-flops, shorts, and t-shirts. As we took our first few sips, I sensed every pair of eyes in the room sizing us up. I didn't have a good feeling. "We walked into the wrong spot," I said to Gina. "We should get out of here."

But just as we stood up to go, somebody grabbed me by the wrist and said with a Jamaican accent, "What's wrong with you, man? You alright?"

I followed the hand gripping me to a Black man with a neatly trimmed beard wearing a dark polo shirt, shorts, and sandals.

"Yeah," I said. "We might just be a little overdressed."

"Hey, don't worry about nothing, Grant," he said and flashed me a policeman's badge. "There's four of us in here. It might look sketchy but nobody's going to mess with you. You're good. You enjoy yourself."

The fact that the cop knew my name helped put me at ease. I bought him a drink even though he was on duty—which didn't stop him from drinking it—and we sat back down. All of a sudden, I forgot all about him or the bottle of Red Stripe beer in front of me or the eyes peering at me from the shadows. A voice came over the speakers singing, "Until the philosophy which hold one race superior and another inferior is finally and permanently discredited and abandoned, everywhere is war…"

I went up and got the bartender's attention. "Who the hell is that?" I asked.

"Man, who is that?" he responded, the look on his face some mix of disbelief and disturbed. "You don't know Bob Marley?"

"Yeah, I know Bob Marley. But that's not on his *Legend* album."

"No, mon. It's from *Backside*," he said.

"*Legend* isn't his only album?"

"Boy, are you playing with me?"

I shrugged and shook my head. "Oh my God," he said. "You stay right there. I'll keep the drinks going and you're going to get treated to Bob Marley tonight."

For the next four or five hours, he played one Marley song after another, none of which I'd heard before. This wasn't "I Shot The Sheriff" or "No Woman, No Cry." This was real shit. Here I am in this little Jamaican bar hearing someone put in words all the bullshit me, my cousins, and my family went through in Georgetown. Bullshit no one had ever had the guts to talk about out loud. *Damn*, I thought. *This fool is talking about it! He ain't*

*talkin' about killin' anybody, he's just talking about the bullshit and
what needs to change.*

We stayed until damn near 4:30 in the morning before
stumbling back to the resort. Poor Gina was probably ready to
go after an hour, but for me it was literally a religious experience.
I was ready to change everything. It wasn't just about becoming
a hardcore Bob Marley or reggae fan. I was all in for becoming
a full-blown Rastafarian. I had found my tribe. I spent our last
few days on the island going into every little store and buying
every booklet I could find on Bob, Rastafarianism, all of it.

I made my conversion painfully clear to everyone once we
got back to Sacramento. I had three video documentaries about
Marley that I made everyone watch. I was pretty damn militant
about it. "If you're going to hang out at my house, you've got to
watch these docs or get the fuck out!" I announced. I watched at
least one of them every day. It wasn't long before word got out:
"If you go to BG's, you can't stay there unless you watch one of
those Marley documentaries."

The trade-off is that I always had plenty of spliffs rolled
and ready. I never smoked during my four years at Xavier and I
didn't touch it for most of my rookie year in the NBA, convinced
I'd get bounced if I tested positive for it. (Ed. note: *The rules
aren't that strict but the NBA has considered marijuana a banned
substance since 1983.*) Vets on the team insisted I wouldn't get in
trouble, but I wasn't willing to risk it. Michael Smith, a fellow

rookie power forward, joined me in abstaining. The season was almost over when someone on the team sparked one up and Michael and I finally gave in and joined them. Sure enough, we were both asked to submit urine samples the very next day! I was sure I was on my way to getting booted from the league but nothing happened.

(When the owners and players negotiated a new collective bargaining agreement in 1996, the players tried to argue its benefits to get it off the banned substances list without incriminating ourselves. At one point, one of the union reps said during the negotiations, "I don't know why you shouldn't have it on there, I just know you shouldn't. I mean, I've heard there's some people out there that it helps them sleep, especially when your—uh, their—back be hurting. Or their knees.")

As it turned out, growing dreadlocks was more of a challenge than not passing a drug test. I didn't have any videos or booklets about growing them. I can't recall seeing anyone with them growing up and I had no idea how to start. We didn't know anything about Bob Marley or reggae in Georgetown. I do remember as a kid I didn't comb my hair for a while once and it knotted up. "What is this?" I remember thinking as I tried to work out the knot. But that was the extent of my knowledge. Kinked-up hair like that was associated with Buckwheat, a poor Black kid with a jacked-up afro in the *Our Gang* TV comedy series. There was nothing about Buckwheat any of us wanted to replicate.

Attempts to get the dreads going myself didn't really work and there wasn't a place in Sacramento back then that did them, so I made a trip to Telegraph Avenue in Oakland, a Black culture mecca a few blocks from the Cal Berkeley campus. While I was there I went to Zebra, a tattoo and piercing joint, and got a Bob Marley tattoo on my right shoulder.

People who hadn't been to my house asked, "Why did you get that?"

I reacted the same way the Jamaican bartender did when I asked him, "Who is that?"

"Shoot, Bob Marley is all that," I told everyone. "You might want to listen to him, man. You might want to put a little bit of that in your life."

I could see the thought bubble over their heads—"Oh shit, this motherfucker is crazy!"—but I didn't care. I knew every word of the documentary and damn near every lyric the man ever wrote. When I say everybody who hung out at the house had to watch it, I mean if there was someone new *everybody* in the house had to watch with them. Watching a video for free weed was a reasonable trade-off so people still came over, but Jermaine thought I'd lost my damn mind and Chuck was worried.

"This is bad," they said.

But Gina, in the first of many examples that she was my ride-or-die girl, would say, "Hey, he likes the Rastas. Leave him alone."

My mom came out to visit and shared Jermaine and Chuck's concern. It wasn't as if I had given up on traditional church. I had found a Methodist pastor in Sacramento that I liked. I wasn't an every-Sunday churchgoer, but I'd attend now and then. But the Rasta way was top of mind. My mom called and told the pastor about my fixation on all things Rastafari and he agreed to meet with us in his chambers.

"You like to fish, right?" he asked.

"Yes," I said.

"And you eat fish, yes?"

"Yes."

"Do you eat the whole fish?"

"Sure."

"Even the bones?"

"No, not the bones."

"Okay. With Rastafarianism, there's some good qualities, things that are good to follow, but there are parts you might want to spit out."

The pastor knew what he was doing. If he had come at me hard about dropping my belief in Rastafarianism, I probably would've felt pressured and defended my interest in it. It wasn't that I rejected what I had learned growing up in Baptist and

Methodist churches; after all, Rastafarianism is a form of Christianity, it just believes in the teachings of only the Old Testament and rejects the Bible's New Testament. More than anything, Rastafarianism spoke to me because it addressed issues such as equality between races and pride in being Black. It offered a view of the world in which I had a reason to stand up for myself, the same way N.W.A. had. The lyrics from Marley's "War," were what was I looking for from my spirituality:

"That until the basic human rights are equally guaranteed to all without regard to race, dis a war."

My research also had turned up aspects of Rastafarianism that didn't work for me, especially that the late Ethiopian emperor Haile Selassie was from the line of Judah, Christ reincarnated. I just couldn't square that with what I'd learned in church growing up. As obsessed with Rasta as I might've seemed, I wasn't totally blinded by it. It had its appeal but it wasn't perfect.

The pastor essentially allowed me to go à la carte with my spirituality—take the parts that worked for me from the various faiths and put them together.

As for the dreads, I couldn't really figure out the trick to growing them until I moved to Portland to play for the Trail Blazers. Chuck came back from playing overseas for a season with them and showed me how he had learned to do it himself.

One of the perks to being an NBA player is if you have a passion for something, you're going to get a chance to experience it in a way few people can. When Bob Marley's son, Ziggy, came through Portland on tour with his band, Ziggy Marley and the Melody Makers, they contacted the Blazers and invited me to their show.

I'm not sure who was more starstruck, them of me or me of them. After the concert, they sent someone to invite Gina and me onto their tour bus. I was fidgety as hell, blown away by the fact that I was hanging with the sons—Ziggy and Stephen—and daughters—Cedella and Sharon—of the man whose work and philosophy I idolized.

"Grant, calm down, mon!" Ziggy said at one point. "Let us see the picture of Daddy." He meant my tattoo of Bob. "You know people in the islands think you're a Marley," Ziggy said.

I couldn't keep the smile off my face. While we sat there, they allowed a few select fans onto the bus for a quick meet-and-greet. It made me think even more highly of them, because they did it out of genuine gratitude for the people who supported their music. "We're just humans," Ziggy said. "We appreciate that people have an admiration for what we do."

While I revered the Marley family, I couldn't come close to how fanned out the people who came on the bus were. They were also high as high could be. It actually became a little tiring, because they talked about Bob as if they knew him better than his kids.

"Your dad was the greatest, a prophet," one said. Everybody had a story to tell. "Do you know that your dad also…"

They'd finally say, "Jah Rastafari!" and then stumble off the bus.

But Ziggy and the others were always polite. "Yes, okay, brother, yes," they would say, no matter how whack the story was. They drew the line at allowing the visitors to misquote scripture or suggest some interpretation they considered incorrect. They had every line memorized. "Wait, wait, mon, you're not right, here's what it says," and they'd grab a Bible and flip to the quoted piece of scripture and then read it.

Jermaine loved that my fascination with Marley became well-known to NBA fans. There was a spot on the backside of the arena where they let fans wait to get autographs from us on our way to our cars. It never failed that at least two or three fans would hand me a ganja-related goodie bag. One kid made a pipe that had a terrific painting of Marley on it. Others just gave me bags of weed that Jermaine often confiscated. "Go on, take it," I told him once. "If you start convulsing, I'll let everybody know you're smoking shit and you don't know where it came from," I said.

The trip to Jamaica, the visit to Georgetown that summer, and the news that Amanda was pregnant with my child should've given Gina a pretty clear look at what she was in for with me. On the visit home, Uncle John, the man who put me on the path to becoming an NBA player, was acting really strange. He couldn't sit still and he was paranoid as hell, talking about people looking for him, or coming after him. Gina liked him but he clearly made her nervous. I suspected he was on some kind of substance. My family always has run a little crazy and hot, but nobody was prepared when he pulled out a handgun and started waving it around, shouting, "Motherfuckers are after me, but I'll kill them all!"

Everybody freaked out and scrambled to get away from him. Maybe I should've been afraid, too, but I knew there was no way he'd turn that gun on me. "Uncle John, let me have the gun," I said. He didn't try to keep me away. I got close enough to take it off him and gave it to my mom.

I knew that Uncle John had had a rough go of it over the last year. My Aunt Belinda had left him and he'd lost his house. He had taken up with a White woman who said she'd marry him if he bought her a trailer for them to live in, but he was just scraping by as it was. As he explained all this, I happened to have about $2,200 in my pocket.

"If that's going to make you happy, here ya go," I said and handed him the wad of cash.

All I know for sure after that is he put the trailer in her name and that's where he died from a gunshot to the head later that summer. There were three people there when it happened—the woman, Uncle John, and a Black dude with red hair named

Chick. The woman apparently had gone back on her word after they bought the trailer, hadn't married him, and eventually kicked him out. I don't know why he was there that day, just as I don't know why Chick was there. Chick and the woman claim he put the gun to his head and pulled the trigger. The police investigation lasted a day or two before they agreed with that scenario, ruling it a suicide. Uncle John was down on his luck, to be sure, but no one in our family, least of all me, believes he killed himself.

There were two things Uncle John loved after his kids: Mike Tyson and me being in the NBA. "They're already beat when they touch gloves!" he said of Tyson's opponents. Without Uncle John, I never would have made it to the NBA. I was devastated thinking, *What if…? What if I had brought him out to Sacramento with me? What if I hadn't given him the money? What if I'd looked deeper into why he was acting so strange?*

What I didn't know is that I was just getting started on my pile of regrets.

As a rookie, outside of my fling with Amanda, I was pretty much on lockdown when it came to messing around; and I'd like to think even that wouldn't have happened if we'd landed as planned in Sacramento. Between falling in love with Gina and wanting to make the Kings' fans who booed and talked shit about me eat their words, I didn't have time for a whole lot else. Besides, making the jump to an 82-game season after playing

117 spread out over four years in college was no joke, especially for someone who made it on out-working the competition. Doing all that as a rookie without having had a proper training camp put me in catch-up mode all year.

I came off the bench for 21 of our first 23 first games, but two days after Christmas, following a blowout loss to the Seattle SuperSonics, I was put in the starting lineup the next night for a one-point win over the Blazers(!), started the rest of the season, and made the All-Rookie first team. It took whatever energy I had left to find ways to hang with Gina and not get caught; and on the road we'd check in to a hotel and I wouldn't even unpack my stuff, I'd just fall into bed and go to sleep.

Looking back, I wasn't prepared for what the NBA threw at me. Not on the court or off it. If I had a little more experience dealing with the temptations of being a young millionaire athlete, or if Gina and I had met at some other point in my life, maybe I would've done a better job of honoring what she meant to me. What she did for me.

Then again, maybe not.

Not the birth of my first son, Amani, to Amanda right before my second season in the NBA started, nor Gina being pregnant with my second son, Elijah, due in March, did anything to discourage me from exploring my options, which were plentiful. I knew my way around the league now, both on and off the court, so on the road I started hitting the hot spots with my teammates.

I'd never felt more like a rock star than the first preseason game of my second year in the league, when we went to play the expansion Vancouver Grizzlies at their arena in British Columbia. Maybe I hadn't experienced that as a rookie because at home Gina and I couldn't really go out a lot for fear of our relationship being discovered. The Kings also weren't very good, so it's not as if everybody in Sacramento was exactly crazy about us, either. All I know is right around the time Gina and I started to talk about getting married, this door opened to another world, a world that had me thinking, "Am I getting married too soon?"

Just like the fog-diverted flight to Oakland led to my hook-up with Amanda, being on the first NBA team to play in Vancouver, B.C., led to another act of unfaithfulness to Gina. Ever felt like the normal rules don't apply to you when you're in a foreign country? That's how I felt when we went to play the expansion Grizzlies in their first-ever preseason game. Flying in is pretty dramatic, coming up over a ridge and suddenly seeing the city all lit up next to the water with the mountains in the background. It's a melting pot of a city with all sorts of cultures. It was easy to forget that we were there on a work trip. Or that I had a girlfriend at home and was in court fighting for custody of a son mothered by a different woman. That was all real-life stuff happening back in the United States. This was a different world.

Six or seven of us went out as soon as we dropped our bags at the hotel to a club called Level 5. We walked in and everyone turned their heads. "Oh, my God, it's the Grizzlies!" someone shouted and everybody started cheering. Finally somebody else said, "No, it's the Sacramento Kings." That only prompted another cheer to go up. It was as if they were just excited to have NBA players coming to their city and hanging out in their club, and I guess they were. None of us were prepared for that. We felt like honored guests.

That's how I met Monica.

I noticed her right away. Long, black hair. Asian features. Carried herself noticeably different than everybody else. I watched as guy after guy in the club approached her and she would just turn her head. I decided to call it a night, but I had to go by her on my way to the door, so I said, "Hi."

She didn't turn her head. She looked at me. "Are you leaving?"

"Yeah," I said. "What are you doing?"

"Nothing," she said.

I sat down. We talked. And then we ended up going back to the hotel. I had no intention of hurting Gina. Somehow, the fact that Monica was so different made it acceptable in my head. She was different from anybody I'd ever met before—her dad was Chinese-Brazilian and her mom was a native Brazilian. She was very attentive right from the start, asking me if I would like a drink. Aggressive. I was hooked. Different girl, different country… different rules, right? Suddenly I was looking for every possible excuse to make a trip to Vancouver. EA Sports, which was originally based there, proved to be a perfect one. I flew up on the premise that I had to test games or meet with them about using my likeness and would grab a couple of brochures to take home with me.

Despite that, and as crazy as it sounds, I couldn't imagine my life without Gina. It's why, with her nearly ready to pop with Elijah, we went to the Sacramento Justice of the Peace over the NBA's February All-Star break and got married. I wanted what I wanted (Monica) but didn't want to lose what I had (Gina). Young buck mentality. Young, dumb, immature buck mentality.

One of the good traits I inherited is that no matter what happens, family sticks together. It's why I was adamant that I would be part of Amani's life. I don't know if Amanda really didn't want that or she was upset with me, but she didn't make it easy. She told the courts that I wasn't fit to be a parent, even though I'd taken care of a sister 11 years younger than me growing up and had Elijah at home. In order to prove I deserved joint custody, I had to drive from Sacramento to Benicia to have my ability to take care of Amani evaluated. Amanda would drop him off and then a man and woman would observe me for an hour with him as I fed him and changed his diaper. After the third visit, they finally said, "We don't know why you're here. You've clearly handled kids before."

I told them what I'd really like to do is bring Elijah with me so he and Amani could meet. They approved of the idea and suggested I bring Gina with me.

That, though, turned out to be an absolute sin for Amanda. What I didn't know is that whenever she dropped off Amani, she would park around the corner and watch the house. So when we brought Elijah down to meet Amani, she saw Gina go in with me and that set her off. She tried to get the couple fired and I thought she'd find a way to keep me from seeing Amani, but we eventually worked everything out. Or at least found a way to keep the hurt feelings at a manageable simmer.

Gina, meanwhile, showered as much attention on Amani as she did Elijah. She didn't see him as the son of a rival but simply a sweet, slightly scared little boy. How she handled that situation, the unconditional love she showed Amani, is one more stinging reminder that I let someone truly special get away.

Life on the court started getting difficult as well my third year in Sacramento. I'd had surgery to repair a meniscus tear in my right knee in college, but that was barely a blip on my athletic radar. Five games into the 1996–97 season, I suffered a hairline fracture in my femur. It felt like a pulled groin that just wouldn't go away. I applied low-level ultrasound to my leg every night in hopes of speeding up the healing process. It took four months for it to improve enough for me to play. Once the doctors assured me my leg would not fail, that's all I needed to hear. I had ample reason to sit out the entire season, but I wanted to play—with a career that didn't start until my senior year in high school, the thrill of putting on a uniform and simply getting to compete was still fresh. There was also the business of being an NBA player.

I had a three-year opt-out clause in my 13-year, $29 million rookie contract, meaning I could become a free agent that summer. There wasn't anything that I didn't like about the city or the team; we had a relatively young roster and liked to hang out together. I became good friends with someone whose early years in the game were completely opposite to mine: Bobby Hurley.

The Hurley name was big in the New Jersey/New York area; playing for his dad, Bob Hurley, Sr., at St. Anthony's High School, Bobby won four parochial state titles. Then he went to Duke and led them to back-to-back NCAA titles. Drafted seventh overall by the Kings a year ahead of me, he had a near-fatal car accident that should've ended his career. It blew out a tendon in his knee; collapsed his lungs; broke his shoulder, ribs, and a couple vertebrae; and nearly ripped his face off. He never thought twice about not playing again. I wouldn't have, either. That he made it back to play four more seasons is amazing, but he was never the same.

One of my favorite memories is shooting dice with Hurley and center Olden Polynice in the hallway of the team hotel whenever we were on the road. Hurley and O.P. would get into an argument, the 6-foot Jersey kid vs. the 7-foot Haitian from the Bronx, and accuse each other of cheating. We were constantly having to pull them apart. It was entertaining as hell.

As a team, though, we seemed to be headed in the wrong direction. My rookie year we narrowly missed making the playoffs with a 39–43 record. That same record the next year was good enough to land the last spot in the Western Conference, earning us the right to face tough guy George Karl and the SuperSonics, who beat us in a best-of-five series, 3–1. That had everyone in Sacramento excited about the following season, but we killed that enthusiasm pretty quick with a 7–14 start. We never made it back to .500, though we got close (28–32) before losing 13 of our next 14 games. Final record: 34–48. As bad as that sounds, it was only two losses worse than the Los Angeles Clippers, who grabbed the last playoff spot despite not having a single All-Star on their roster. This was back when being worse than the Clippers was a kiss of death—and so it was for St. Jean, who was fired and replaced by his assistant, Eddie Jordan, with 15 games left.

All of that made it seem like a good time to see what else might be out there for me. The amazement and thrill of just being in the NBA had worn off. Now that I'd made it, I wanted to do something special. The Kings hadn't had a winning season for 14 consecutive years and there were no signs of that streak ending.

I did enough in the final weeks of the season to prove I was as good as I had been before the injury. I started slow but averaged 15.1 points and 8.5 rebounds over an eight-game stretch near the very end. That was actually better than what I had averaged my first two years overall.

Mark, my agent, started making calls. As it turned out, the next team up the coast was looking to make some changes as well. When Mark told me the Portland Trail Blazers were very interested, I became very interested in them. It occurred to me that over my first three years in the league, I'd never had a bad game against the Blazers. That had not escaped their attention.

But if I thought the year I'd had in Sacramento was full of personal drama off the court and my body working against me on it, I was in for a much more stressful one, in every way, in Portland.

chapter 6

Playing with Secrets

There was one problem with my desire to join the Blazers and their interest in signing me: they didn't have any room on their roster or on their payroll. Not unless they were willing to say goodbye not just to one but a couple of the fans' favorite players.

They were.

Mark would not have let me opt out of my contract with the Kings unless he knew he could get me a better deal than the $26 million over 10 years I still had coming to me. The Blazers did more than that—their six-year, $56 million offer made me the second-highest paid player on the team, just behind point guard Kenny Anderson. For one of the few times in my career, I felt like someone was betting on me.

To do that, though, they had to cash in their chips on a power forward Blazers fans loved: Cliff Robinson. (Ed. note: *"Uncle Cliffy," as he was known, was exactly the kind of player Trail*

Blazers fans see not just as one of their own but one of them—the basketball version of a lumberjack, the unassuming flannel-collared, work-booted man's man who fells the mighty through sheer, relentless determination. Drafted by the Blazers in the second round of the 1990 draft, Cliff was deep into his sixth season before he missed a game. His 461 consecutive appearances is still a franchise record. He helped the Blazers go to the conference finals three years in a row and reach the Finals twice. He earned his nickname with a celebratory dance on the court after the Blazers beat the Utah Jazz in the 1992 conference finals to take a commanding 3–1 lead in the best-of-seven series. When asked about the dance afterward, he called it the "Uncle Cliffy."

He was also an unorthodox player and people in Portland like things that are a little weird or different. Cliff, at 6'10" and 228 pounds, was the early prototype of a "stretch 4" in today's game, a power forward who can rebound and defend against bigger players but offensively plays as much or more on the perimeter as he does around the basket. Coach Rick Adelman used him at three different positions—small forward, power forward, and center—and Cliff did whatever was needed wherever he was needed. He was recognized as the league's Sixth Man of the Year in 1993 and an All-Star in 1994.)

I wasn't the only one trying to replace a hometown favorite. Bob Whitsitt, after being named 1994 Executive of the Year for building the Seattle SuperSonics into the best team in the West, was hired away by owner and Microsoft billionaire Paul

Allen to replace Geoff Petrie, known as "The Original Blazer." If you want to do something to make people in Portland mad, import something from Seattle. To really make them mad, import something from Seattle to replace something homegrown in Portland. (Ed. note: *The first draft pick in the team's history, Petrie won NBA co-Rookie of the Year and was a two-time All-Star, spending his entire six-year playing career with the Blazers. In 1985, he rejoined the franchise as a color commentator for their radio broadcasts before moving into the front office.*)

I learned this pretty quickly about Blazers' fans: they don't let just anybody into their hearts, but once they do let you in, you're in for good. Geoff and the players who made their team the one to beat for three years in the Western Conference had lifetime passes. Bob, on the other hand, was seen as the hatchet man getting rid of dudes who gave their sweat and blood to make the Blazers—and thereby Portland—respected: Jerome Kersey, Clyde Drexler, Buck Williams, Terry Porter, and Kevin Duckworth. Cliff was the last holdover of the nucleus that made those two runs to the Finals and created what is known among Blazers' fans as "The Rip City Revival."

That was the cat I was replacing, along with Chris Dudley, who wasn't part of the group that went to the Finals but, like Cliff, was a workhorse who rarely missed a game or gave less than all-out effort. (Ed. note: *Anyone who ever saw his ungainly free-throw-shooting form would say he had that touch of odd that*

Portlanders love, too.) The Blazers traded Dudley to the New York Knicks at the start of training camp, essentially so they could afford to pay me.

Now imagine trying to make good on all that with one arm and a wife who didn't want to move.

The day we flew up for our first visit to Portland—Gina and Elijah went with me—it was 100 degrees and sunny in Sacramento and 60 degrees and rainy in Portland. "You get to go to LA and Miami and places like that," she said, "while I'm going to be back here in the rain all the time."

Fair point. Here it was, summertime, and yet it was a nasty bone-chilling wet day. *Oh, man,* I thought. *I don't know if we can do this.* But then Mark presented us the terms of the contract and I looked at Gina and said, "Yeah, we can do this."

I also couldn't see letting cold rain stop me from playing for a team as loaded with talent as the Blazers. I had already been paying attention to the moves they were making my last year in Sacramento. They had drafted a young power forward straight out of high school, Jermaine O'Neal, and traded for another young power forward/center, Rasheed Wallace, along with a young shooting guard, Isaiah "JR" Rider. They also had another power forward from Ohio, Gary Trent, and the great Lithuanian center Arvydas Sabonis, who they had drafted 12 years earlier. He had finally decided to come to the NBA after tearing up the European leagues and his Achilles tendon. He didn't move very well, but at

7'3" and nearly 300 pounds with a three-point shooting touch and passing skills as good as any big man in the game, he was still a force. Trader Bob was putting together something special.

That's also a lot of talented big men, but I saw myself fitting in somehow—as a big small forward, a power forward, or even as a center. I didn't care where. I was excited to figure it out.

I was especially looking forward to playing with Rasheed, or "Sheed," as most people call him. We'd been battling since he came into the league with the Washington Bullets a year after me. We talked trash and tried to dunk on each other all game long every time we faced each other. I just thought he was the coolest cat and I loved his game.

It took most of the summer to work out the deal. Some of it was because the Blazers had to figure out some other moves to make everything work financially. I wanted to make a good first impression whenever the time came to move to Portland, so I made sure to stay in shape while we were still in Sacramento. That meant getting in the regular run at the Salvation Army. That's where it happened. I don't remember exactly how or when I did it, but I did something that left my shoulder feeling sore and weak. Now, I had yet to take a physical or sign my new deal with the Blazers. My whole focus became passing the physical. If they had asked for an MRI on my shoulder at that point, I'm sure they would've said, "What the fuck is this?" But they didn't call for one because I'd never had any shoulder problems. They were more concerned about my knees and legs.

What worried me the most is that I knew they'd have me bench press some amount of weight as part of the physical—I don't know what they do now but it was pretty standard back then. Normally, that would have been a piece of cake, but I had no idea what they'd ask me to lift and if my shoulder would give out. I didn't want to test it before that and risk doing more damage or really messing it up. Instead, I arranged to get a cortisone shot the day before the physical. Then, mentally, all I thought about was getting that bar down to my chest and back up again. I fired off three reps real quick—bop-bop-bop—until they said, "Okay, good. Good."

It didn't stay good, though. Right out of the gate, in one of my first pick-up runs in Portland, boom! My right arm got pulled back and I felt something pop. I was playing at Club Sport, a fitness center across the street from the Blazers' headquarters. I walked over and talked to the team athletic trainer, Jay Jensen. He examined my shoulder and sent me directly to the hospital to get an MRI.

When I came in the next day, he said, "You're going to be out six to eight months."

"What?" I asked.

"You tore your labrum. Sometimes people get a tear in that thing and you can shave it down and maybe just put a suture in it, but yours is really torn up. They're going to have to drill down and put dissolvable screws in it."

And I'm thinking: *Holy shit! And I just signed here?* I knew the fans were pissed about Cliff, Chris, and the rest of the Blazers who had been shipped out to make room for me, Sheed, Jermaine, and JR. I also knew how they'd feel about a new kid with a big-ass contract who can't play because of a shoulder injury. Probably a lot like the Kings' fans felt about an unknown rookie who had just been made a lottery pick and doesn't show up for training camp. This, though, meant missing the entire season.

"Jay, if I don't play, this city will never respect me," I said. "I don't care how much I do, they'll never respect me. What can you do to help me get through this?"

"There's no way you can play with that," he said.

"I have to."

Jay stared at me. I think it took him a beat to see that I was serious about playing, not just with a bad shoulder, but a bad shooting shoulder. (I'm right-hand dominant.) "Well, you're allowed a certain amount of cortisone shots," he said. "And you can take anti-inflammatories, but no painkillers or anything like that."

Jay and I became best friends because I spent more time with him than anybody else. He monitored everything and wouldn't let me take any kind of opioid or nerve-numbing medication, even though I'm sure he knew it would've given me some relief.

After every game he'd strap bags of ice to my shoulder and set me up with a TENS unit (transcutaneous electrical nerve stimulator) at home to create natural endorphins to dull the ache. Some nights I'd be up all night, tossing and turning, crying because the throbbing pain just wouldn't subside. He allowed me a cortisone shot twice over the course of the season and both times I had a couple days of feeling pretty good before they wore off. Going up and down in planes was particularly bad. I don't know if it was the change in altitude or cabin pressure, but my shoulder would throb and I'd have to grip the arm rest and clench my teeth until we leveled off or landed.

It's amazing what someone 25 years old and in the prime of his athletic life can make his body endure, especially if his pride is on the line. I played 61 of 82 regular-season games (starting 49) and after almost every one of them Jay said, "You probably need to take care of that now."

My answer was always the same: "No, Jay, I'm going to play through it."

I didn't just play, I played like someone mad at the world. I was actually mad at myself, but I made everyone I played against—in practices and games—pay the price.

My numbers were respectable—31.5 minutes a game, 12.1 points, and 9.1 rebounds, while shooting better than 50 percent. (Did I mention the torn labrum was in my shooting shoulder?) I couldn't lift weights or do anything else that might irritate it.

Some games the adrenalin and the anti-inflammatories would kick in just right and I felt good. There were other nights when I focused on positioning myself so I could do my job—defend and rebound—without involving my right shoulder.

We finished with a slightly worse record than the year before—46–36 instead of 49–33—but only dropped one spot in the playoff seeding, from fifth to sixth. That earned us a first-round matchup with the Los Angeles Lakers. These were not the Phil-Kobe-Shaq Lakers yet—Kobe was still coming off the bench as a second-year player—but they were still pretty damn good. It was pretty much The Shaq Show. If anyone in the league could hold his own against Shaq it was Sabonis, because he had the size (7'3", 275 pounds), could finish with either hand around the basket, and could pull Shaq away from the basket with his jump shot and sweet passing.

But this was Shaq in his physical prime, 25 years old. Sabas was 33 with two Achilles tendon surgeries. Every game went pretty much the same way: we'd start with Sabas guarding Shaq one-on-one, he'd get in foul trouble, we'd have to double-team Shaq to keep our whole front line from fouling out, which would leave another Laker open for wide-open shots. We were still figuring out how we wanted to play at both ends of the court and the playoffs aren't a good place to do that. We nearly stole the first game in L.A., losing 104–102, and we won Game 3 in Portland, but a team with enough talent to have Kobe Bryant coming off the bench is going to be tough to beat. Besides, while Lakers coach Del Harris might not have been starting Kobe, he made sure to have him on the floor when it mattered most—at the end of every game.

I had a good series, but I also had a motivational tank that was full, thanks to Jerry West cursing me out and threatening to make sure I never wore an NBA uniform. I can't blame him for feeling the way he did—I bombed my workout—and he's a legend so I never did anything to embarrass or confront him, but whenever I saw him I made sure he saw me. The Lakers knocked us out in four games, but all my averages went up (33.8 minutes, 13.3 points, 10.8 rebounds, 52.8 percent shooting) from the regular season, which is not what happened in Sacramento when I had two healthy shoulders.

There was one other reason that fueled the reckless, relentless way I played that entire season: I had to keep a big secret and the court was the one place I could blow off the pressure I felt because of it.

And I'm not talking about my shoulder.

When I realized we were about to move to Portland, I called Monica and ended it. She took it well. "That's fine," she said. "I understand." Then, two weeks later, she called me back. "I just found out," she said. "I'm pregnant."

So much for a clean break. As much as I wished I could just put our relationship firmly behind me, I didn't think it would be right to tell her what to do with the baby. That, I felt, had to be her decision. "What do you think you want to do?" I asked.

"I don't know," she said.

"Well, let me know when you know."

A few weeks after we moved to Portland, Gina said, "Guess what?"

"What?"

"We're having another baby."

That was one more reason to play—or, rather, not to have surgery and spend the next six months sitting at home waiting for my shoulder to heal. By now, my conscience was getting the better of me. Gina was growing up right in front of me, turning into a sophisticated woman, and now I had jeopardized what we had and I didn't know how any of it was going to work out. She wanted more of my time than I was willing to give because I felt guilty that there was a chance I might put her in another situation exactly like I had with Amanda. Only this time I didn't even have the excuse that we hadn't started messing around yet or were truly a couple. I need to chill out, I thought, before I end up losing her—if I haven't already.

Being a maniac going after every rebound and getting wild-eyed in every opponent's face endeared me to Blazers' fans, even if they didn't know what was fueling it. It even earned me a nickname: Rasta Monsta. I'd always played with an edge, but up until now it had always been about proving someone who had doubted me wrong. This was about letting go of the anger, fear, and frustration I felt about the predicament I'd created. As much as my shoulder hurt, I convinced myself that having surgery and then sitting around with all that guilt would've driven me crazier.

Just when I needed mental relief from the constant ache in my shoulder and darkness in my soul, something really special happened. Gina convinced me to attend a charity fashion show put on to support the local children's hospital. There was a meet-and-greet party afterward. That's where I met Miguel Reyes, a former school teacher and future confidant. There was something about Miguel that triggered my curiosity and he told me his story. His mother was a Native American and his dad was Mexican. He had a measured way of talking and a careful way of listening that captivated me. Jovita, his daughter and one of the runway models, was battling leukemia.

I was in the process of creating a foundation to help families with terminally ill children. Brian Berger, who was part of the Blazers' public relations staff, was helping me and introduced me to Lauren Forman, who became my foundation director. So I gave Miguel and his wife, Cassandra, my number and told them to call me, in part because I thought my foundation could help them, but also because I got such a good vibe from talking to them.

We got to know each other over the following months. Then, one night, I had just walked off the court after a game when

Berger got a message to me that Jovita was in the hospital and they weren't sure she would make it through the night. I ran in to the locker room and threw my sweats on over my uniform and rushed to the hospital.

When I saw Miguel I asked, "Did she—?"

"No," he said. "She's fighting. She's hanging on."

Jovita survived that night, but at one point while we were waiting for the crisis to pass, Miguel turned to me and said, "I'm having trouble being a father to my son because all my attention is on my daughter right now. I'd really appreciate it if you would just talk to him, let him know he's not alone."

His son's name was Ramon. I was happy to do it. Helping the Reyes family allowed me to forget about my own problems. It became a daily routine. Jermaine and Chuck would go down to their house and kick it with Ramon when we were on the road or had a game; if I had practice, they'd bring him back to my place so we could hang out afterward. He'd talk about his sister, how he was praying she'd get well. That's a lot for a kid in 10th grade to carry and it felt good to give him an outlet to talk about it.

I knew all about the burden of keeping a secret. I was living it. The tears and sleepless nights weren't all about my shoulder. Monica had decided she was having the baby. I was of the mind, as I had been with Amani, that no matter what the circumstances, I was not going to have any kid of mine grow up without having me in his life. Which meant at some point I was going to have to

181

tell Gina. I'd lie in bed, staring at the ceiling, thinking, "I messed up. I messed this all up. I've got a beautiful woman who loves me. I've got a son with her and another one on the way. And all of it could be gone."

I couldn't tell anybody close to me about Monica because as soon as Gina found out, she'd feel betrayed by anyone who knew and hadn't told her. When the bomb dropped, I didn't want anyone else to be in the blast radius.

Berger saw how the Reyes family responded to me and how much it meant to me to spend time with them. He suggested we go see a kid named Dash who had terminal brain cancer. "Okay," I said. We drove out to his house one day, me in the car with ice packs still strapped to my knees and shoulder from practice. I mentally prepared myself to meet a kid in a wheelchair or in a bed, barely able to move or talk.

We rolled down to his house and he came running out the front door to meet us. "Hey, what's up?" I said to cover my surprise. "How you doin', Dash?"

"I'm good, man," said the kid with terminal brain cancer. The kid's spirit blew me away. We ended up shooting hoops in his driveway and talking. Before we left, I said, "Why don't I come back and we can go to the movies or bowling or something?"

I could tell by the look on the faces of his parents—Dave and Robin—that they wished I hadn't said that, mainly because they didn't believe I meant it. They told me as much later. As much as they appreciated that I came down to see Dash, they didn't want him getting his hopes up that it would happen again. "We just wanted him to cherish that it happened once," they said.

But after hanging with Dash, I just couldn't imagine going on with my life and having them go on with theirs. So, a couple of weeks later, Berger arranged for me to take Dash and some of his friends to a bowling alley. We had a blast. Many years later, a couple of those kids approached me as adults. "We went to the bowling alley with you when Dash was sick," they said. What they didn't know—maybe couldn't know—is that they and Dash did as much or more to lift my spirits at the time. It also helped remind me that doing something with somebody, even something as simple as a trip to a bowling alley, can create really special memories.

Jovita and Dash, in their way, inspired and gave me perspective on my circumstances. As much as I had complicated my life and as torn up as I felt about it, I was an adult who had created my own problems and had a chance to make things right. They were just kids dealt a bad hand through no fault of their own and were making the best of it. (Their example would help me even more after I was diagnosed with PD.) For now, it made me feel better about myself as a human being. And any time I questioned why God had let me get to this place in my life, I'd think of them and how they weren't even getting the chance to have half the life I'd had. As a young parent, I'd think about my kids and not just what Dash and Jovita's parents were going through, but all the parents I'd see in the hospital's pediatric ward. They had this hopeless, resigned look, not knowing if their kid would still be alive the next week and I'd think, *I don't know how to help you!* And I'd imagine what it would be like to switch places with them. And all that would straighten me up quick.

The better I got to know Jovita's and Dash's parents, the more I thought about their reaction when it got out that I was the father of two kids born to different mothers about a month apart. I had no intention of it getting out, but I also knew the ease with which gossip got around small towns. Would the parents then be upset that I'd spent time with their kids? That I befriended them? That I allowed them to look up to me? It was going to make me look bad when it got out, but I didn't want it to make anyone else look bad, especially anyone who might've spoken up for me as a good guy. I didn't want any of them waking up one morning and reading about me in the newspaper and wondering, "What is going on?"

I'm pretty good about having a hard conversation when I think it needs to be had. Miguel was the first person I told. That sense I had of him being someone special the first time I saw him proved to be accurate. He had that school teacher's way of slipping you bits of wisdom in increments just big enough for the moment. He never over-did it or under-did it. And that's how he handled me telling him about Monica.

"Hey, brother, we get down but we got to get back up," he said. "We all do. I have to, my son, you have to. I know you're not a man who abandons his kids. So you need to be there for Gina, your son, *and* your other son. You have to be there for them all." That wouldn't be the last time we talked about it. Several times over the course of the season I'd call Miguel, wracked with guilt and shame, and he'd calm me down.

When I approached Robin and Dave and said, "Soooo, this is what's going on in my life," they were just as understanding. I thought they might say, "Don't come around my son no more."

Instead, they said, "Hey, everybody makes mistakes. There's nothing we could find out about you, Brian, that would change the way we feel about you. We just want to know if you're okay."

"I'm okay," I told them. "You know, I was worried. I didn't know if you guys would want me to still come around."

"No, Brian," they said, "you've been a blessing."

There was one more person I had to tell: Dick Inukai, the owner of several local car dealerships. It turned out to be the hardest.

Dick happened to live right up the street from me, so I'd think of him every time I pulled into my driveway in the Ford truck he had loaned me for promotional purposes. I finally walked over to his house and knocked on the door. When he answered I said, "Sir, can I talk to you for a minute?"

He invited me in and we sat down. "What's on your mind, Brian?" he asked.

"Well," I said, "I don't know if I should be driving your car."

That caught him off-guard. Dick thought there must be something wrong with the truck. "Why? Did we do something wrong?"

"No, it's not what you did. It's what I did. I think you need to know that I had an extramarital affair and she ended up getting pregnant and my wife is pregnant, too, and I don't know what is going to happen, but I don't want any of this to reflect on you for having loaned me a car."

Dick put his hand on my shoulder and looked at me. "Son, I wouldn't want anybody but you to drive our car," he said. "I know how hard this must have been for you."

His kindness and forgiveness opened up the floodgates. "It was," I choked out through my tears.

"No, hey, hey," he said. "We want you to represent us."

So everyone I felt had to know now knew. I didn't want any publicity about my visits to Dash or Jovita or my foundation because I didn't want to make it seem I was going out of my way for people to see me as a good guy. So Berger and I kept all of it to ourselves until the parents of one of Dash's friends called the local paper, *The Oregonian*, and basically said, "You write all these negative articles about the Blazers. Here's a good one. Brian Grant's been coming down and seeing a young, terminally ill kid.

He took him and my kids bowling. You guys might want to try writing about that."

The paper and every other news outlet in the area swooped in to cover the story. I told Robin and Dave that a bunch of reporters had asked me if they could interview them but that they didn't have to do any of it. A part of me hoped they wouldn't but I didn't consider it my place to tell them what they should do. Anyway, they agreed to talk about Dash and me. I never asked them why. My guess is they thought bringing awareness to what Dash was fighting would help him. Sharing their story probably helped them, too.

The next time I saw Dash, he was moving slower because of the medication he had to take for the pain. It also prevented him from being able to control his farts. We started laughing and then I started cutting them. "I can't help it," I said. "You gave me permission to start up, too."

I got through the season, but Dash didn't. A few weeks later, he took a turn for the worse and had to go back to the children's hospital. He couldn't speak and his eyes were shut. I said a prayer with his parents and kissed each one of them—Dash, Robin, and Dave—before I left. It was the last time I saw Dash alive.

Then I got a call about a teenager from northeast Portland named Woody. He'd obviously heard about my visits, because when I walked into his hospital room he said, "Damn, I must be dying. They done sent Brian Grant." Have to give it to him—he had a sense of humor.

"No, man," I said, laughing. "I just came in to say hi."

My relationship with Woody was different than with Dash. Woody was a teenager fighting leukemia, wanting to do teenager things and frustrated he couldn't. When we hung out it was more grown-up, back-and-forth conversations. As rough as my teenage years might have seemed to me, I couldn't help but see them in a different light after hanging with Woody. He had been through some things a lot tougher than getting bloodied up on a basketball court.

Woody needed a bone marrow transplant, so we put together a drive to find a match at the Blazers' Boys & Girls Club. Nobody supports their own better than the people of Portland. Hundreds showed up to have their blood drawn and tested to see if they were a match.

Also understand this: I was able to do this stuff because I had good people around me. Berger and the Blazers found the kids and helped hook me up with them. They donated their time and energy as much as I did and were as affected by the kids as I was.

The guy I'm most proud of when it came to the marrow drive is my cousin, Jermaine. He would rather jump in a cage with a lion than get stuck with a needle. There are people who don't like needles, but I don't know anyone who freaks out like Jermaine. When we were kids back in Georgetown, we had to go to the health department to get our school immunization shots. He went first. I remember hearing him screaming and an adult voice saying, "Alright, we need more people!" It took a half-dozen people to hold him down and administer the shot.

Volunteers for the marrow drive have blood drawn and it's then tested to see if they're a match for the person who needs an infusion of new bone marrow. Jermaine, as you might guess, wanted no part of it.

"C'mon, Jermaine, we're trying to help Woody," I said.

Jermaine sighed. "I guess I could do it, cousin."

It's fortunate the drive lasted about a week, because it took a couple of tries with Jermaine. He'd walk in, sit down, and then just as they got ready to draw the blood he'd jump up and run out.

Chuck and I finally cornered him. "Hey, man, you're going to have to go through with it this time," we told him.

"Okay, okay," he said. "Just don't grab me."

I don't know if Jermaine hadn't ever had blood drawn before, but after they inserted the needle into his forearm, he grunted and said, "Oh, that wasn't too bad."

We all watched the vial fill up with blood. When they were finished, I said, "Dang, you did it, Jermaine!"

There is a national registry of people willing to donate their bone marrow. We added a ton of Portlanders to the list. We didn't find a match for Woody, but the registry found one for him, and we were able to provide matches for a couple people in other parts of the country.

(Ed. note: *Brian would receive the league's 1999 J. Walter Kennedy Citizenship Award, which recognizes a player for outstanding citizenship and community service.*)

As soon as the season was over, I made plans to end the agony with my shoulder by flying back to Los Angeles to have surgery. Mark, my agent, convinced me to have Neal ElAttrache, the Los Angeles Dodgers team doctor, do the operation. Pitchers and trapeze artists were his specialty, I was told, and those are some pretty valuable shoulders.

Even the surgery wasn't without complications. Something went wrong as they brought me out of anesthesia and I went into respiratory arrest, a Code Blue in hospital terms. I found out about my close call after I woke up back in my room. Every time I had to go under the knife after that—and I did seven more times during my playing career—I rolled into the operating room fearful I wouldn't make it out.

I went home with my arm in a sling prepared to walk into another situation, not knowing what kind of condition I'd be in coming out of it. It was time to give up my other secret.

Monica gave birth to Jonavan in May; less than a month later, Gina had Jaydon. I waited until Gina was back in shape and feeling good about herself before I broke the news. We had been going to church regularly since we moved to Portland and when it came time to finally come clean, I spoke with our pastor first.

"That's going to be a tough one," he said, "but God will get you through it."

We were getting ready for church one Sunday when I sat down on the edge of the bed.

"What are you doing?" she asked. "We're going to be late."

I shook my head. "We're not going to church," I said. "I've got to tell you something. There's something wrong."

She stopped and looked at me. "I've known something's wrong for a long time, but you wouldn't tell me what," she said. "No one would."

"That's because nobody knows," I said.

"Knows what?"

I was breathing hard.

"I was messing around."

"You cheated on me?" She started to cry. My pastor had been oh so right.

"Yeah." I could barely get the words out. "And something else happened."

"What?"

"There's a kid."

I could feel the weight of the secret that I had been carrying for almost a year come off my neck, my back, my head. But another heaviness replaced it almost immediately when Gina fell down on the bedroom floor sobbing. I sat there, looking down at her. I figured she was done with me, for sure. I was willing to give her anything if it would ease what she was feeling. "Baby, whatever you want, the house, I mean, none of this shit means anything to me anymore if it's not going to be with you," I said.

She remained crumpled on the floor, wailing, for what seemed like forever. I knew better than to try to touch her. So I stood there, swallowing hard, shaking my head, hating myself as much as I ever have. Finally, she looked up at me and said, "You're so fucking stupid!"

"I know," I said. "I'm dumb."

I expected her to say something next, like, "Alright, that's it. I'm leaving and I'm taking the kids."

Instead, she said, "I can't leave you because you've got my heart."

That took me over the edge. Of all the reactions I was prepared for and felt I fully deserved, that was not one. Now *my* tears came hard and fast.

chapter 7

Broken, Bloodied, Beloved

My second season in Portland was messed up, too, but this time I wasn't the architect. The collective bargaining agreement between the players and the team owners had expired and coming to terms on a new one did not go well. As a result, the owners locked us (the players) out and the start of the season was postponed indefinitely.

In a lot of ways, it was a blessing in disguise for me. It allowed me to take more time to rehab my shoulder than I probably would have. It also allowed me to learn about all that living in Oregon has to offer—which was a lot. The players on the roster were what first attracted me about moving to Portland, but once I got there I saw in real life things I'd previously only seen in magazines, things that fascinated me. For example, I've loved fishing since I was a kid, but the only kind I'd ever done was off the banks of the Ohio River or a nearby lake—put on your lure or bait, attach a bell to your line, toss it in the water, and wait for the ding-ding-ding that tells you something swallowed your lure, usually a big shallow-water catfish.

Gina and I bought a house with a yard and part of the interior unfinished. The contractor hired a landscaper, who came to me at one point and said the budget for the exterior wouldn't provide a look that was worthy of the house. I immediately suspected he was just trying to jack up the price and my look must've given that away.

"Alright, I'll do it like shit, if that's the way you want it," he said.

I knew by the way he said it he was shooting me straight. "Okay," I said. "Tell me what you think we should do."

And that's how I met my fishing guide, Craig Prunty, and got a beautifully landscaped yard as well. We sat down over a couple of Budweisers to discuss his ideas about what to do with the yard and at some point the conversation drifted to fishing. He invited me to join him on a trip up the Columbia River to the Bonneville Dam, about 40 miles outside of Portland, to fish for sturgeon. The big ones can get to 100 years old, grow nearly 20 feet long, and weigh 1,500 pounds. I'll never forget watching Craig pull in a 10-footer on that first trip—the first of many. We went river fishing for salmon as well and ocean fishing on the Pacific. He opened my eyes to a whole new world and he was the perfect fishing guide for me, because he wasn't coming home until he'd caught something.

He was also the complete outdoorsman, thanks to his dad, who started taking him up to their cabin in the Northwoods, the forest that sits halfway between the ocean and the city, when he was 13. The man knew how to have fun—he'd ride snowmobiles up Mount St. Helens in the winter and four wheelers and motorcycles on the trails and logging roads in the summers. The first time he took me up to his cabin there was about three feet of fresh fallen snow. The lake was not frozen over but blanketed in white. It was so beautiful. Disappearing into the evergreens, breathing in all that pure rain-washed Northwestern air, and frying up fresh-caught fish over a campfire was exactly what I needed after the stress I'd been carrying since we moved north. I ended up buying the cabin across the road from Craig's and a fishing boat that was nearly identical to his.

It felt as if I were finding my sweet spot, off and on the court. Michael Jordan retired, ending the Chicago Bulls' reign over the Eastern Conference, and the NBA in general. The Utah Jazz still had their dynamic duo, power forward Karl Malone and point guard John Stockton, and a great coach in Jerry Sloan, but after two trips to the Finals only to be stopped by Michael and the Bulls, there was a question of just how much they had left. Karl was 35, John was 36, and their third star, Jeff Hornacek was 35. The Lakers had Kobe Bryant and Shaquille O'Neal, but Kobe was still coming off the bench and Phil Jackson was still a year away from coming out of retirement to coach them. The door was wide open for a team to take the throne and we felt as if we had everything we needed.

There have been plenty of negative things said and written about Rasheed Wallace, but I have nothing but respect for him as a teammate and a player. No one had to make a bigger adjustment than Sheed when I came to Portland. They moved him from power forward to small forward, and although he started, his numbers dipped across the board. I don't think it sat well with him at first, because he wasn't getting the same kind of shots; he was taking fewer of them overall and far more of them from 16 feet and out after showing he could kill guys with either hand in the low post. But it forced him to develop his three-point range and that made him even more of a threat. He could take you down low and bust you or step outside and do the same.

Although the lockout shortened the second year to 50 games, we'd added a ton of talent, so our coach, Mike Dunleavy, spent a good part of the year experimenting with his rotations. Four of our five starters were pretty much set: Sabonis at center, me at power forward, JR Rider at shooting guard, and Damon Stoudamire, who we picked up at the trade deadline the year before from the Toronto Raptors, at point guard. Small forward, though, was a merry-go-round. Sheed, Walt Williams (acquired with Damon from the Raptors), and Stacey Augmon (picked up in a January 1997 trade with the Pistons) all got some run at small forward. Nine different guys in all started at least one game and the shuffle wasn't because of injury—we stayed pretty healthy.

JR wasn't always on time for practice or game-day shootarounds, which prompted Mike to take him out of the starting lineup about eight times over the course of the season, but otherwise we were all available pretty much every night. The top nine guys in the rotation all played in 47 or more of our 50 games, including point guard Greg Anthony, another free-agent addition. Greg always came off the bench and his stats wouldn't exactly blow you away, but he was a great leader. He loves to talk; I knew then already he was going to make a great commentator.

The shifting roles and playing time didn't slow us down; if anything, it kept us fresh, which was a huge advantage. Even with reducing the regular season from 82 to 50 games, the time crunch meant the schedule makers had to break some long-standing rules, such as not having teams play more than two nights in a row. All 29 teams had to play three games in three nights several times; we, though, were the only team to win three times in three nights. It helped that the first and third games were at home and the middle one was in Vancouver, which is under an hour of flying time from Portland.

Mike started a different small forward every game—Stacey in the first, Walt in the second, and Sheed in the third—and the minutes leader changed for all three games as well. (JR had the most in the first, Damon in the second, and Sheed in the third.) What made it work is that all of us checked our egos at the door. Despite being the youngest team in the league, we were less worried about proving what we could do individually and instead focused on what we could be as a team. I remember so many times coming back to the bench after hitting a couple of shots and everybody being happy for me. That doesn't happen on every team. We were tight.

Once the playoffs started, Mike found his rotational groove. Sheed locked down the small forward spot the rest of the way. We made short work of our first-round opponent, the Phoenix Suns, sweeping them in three games. Uncle Cliffy was the Suns' leading scorer and their point guard, Jason Kidd, averaged a double-double in points and assists, but we were just deeper in talent and bigger in size. Sabas—our nickname for Sabonis—and I averaged more than nine rebounds each and combined to block four shots a game, but it was our offense that really overwhelmed them. We shot better than 50 percent as a team for the series (52.8), which almost never happens in the playoffs.

For the first time in a long time, I wasn't hurting, mentally or physically, and the Suns decided to key on Sheed. That left Sabas free to work his magic from the high post. He always seemed to be limping but he didn't have to move to whip a perfect behind-the-back or through-the-legs pass to me cutting to the basket for easy buckets. I made 71.9 percent of my shots to average 19.3 points, second only to JR, who was on fire, averaging 20.

That put us up in the second round against the reigning Western Conference champs, the Jazz, and me up against Malone, who had been named league MVP for the regular season for the second time in three years.

Since they had the better regular-season record and were the higher seed, they had home-court advantage and the series started in their arena, the Delta Center. It feels as if the fans are sitting right on top of you and by halftime your ears are ringing from the crowd noise. I never liked playing there. The fans were rude and at times a tad bit racist in their taunts.

What made Karl one of the best power forwards ever is that he was super strong, super physical, and super fast. The only way to slow him down was to get physical with him, but the referees made that hard to do. The first game was a perfect example: Karl nearly fouled out our entire front line while scoring 13 of his 25 points on free throws. At one point, he elbowed me in the face and they called a foul on me. The league office later reviewed the play and fined Karl $10,000 for the incident, but that did nothing to stop me from fouling out after playing only 31 minutes. Sheed had five fouls and Sabonis had four.

Karl wasn't the only Jazz player who had tricks. I was playing in Miami when Stockton set a pick on me and caught me right in the ribs. When I knocked him down later as payback, he jumped right up and said, "I'm still standing!" John, Karl, and Jeff Hornacek were all clever at getting sneaky shots in that the refs couldn't see, but then abruptly stopping or changing direction and getting you to run in to them so that the refs felt they had to blow the whistle. Anyway, Stockton had Damon in foul trouble, too, with five, and they outscored us 30–15 on free throws for a 93–83 win.

We were more mad than disappointed. Despite feeling handcuffed by the refs, we had led going into the fourth quarter, 78–74. That's right—we were outscored 19–5 in the final 12 minutes, including 11–1 on free throws. (Ed. note: *That remains a league playoff record for fewest points scored in a fourth quarter.*)

NBA security and a Utah Jazz fan made sure I had all the motivation I needed for Game 2. The phone rang in my hotel room, waking me up from my pregame nap. It was Horace Balmer, the NBA head of security. "Man, we've got an issue with a young lady and we've got to resolve it," he said.

"Okay, but why are you calling me?" I asked, rubbing my eyes.

"Come on, Grant," he said. "You've got a chance to come clean with this."

I was starting to get mad. "What are you talking about?"

Horace sounded mad, too. "Alright, you want to do it the hard way? We can do it the hard way."

"I'm calling my agent."

Mark and I called Horace back. "Mark, I don't know this girl," I said to both of them.

"Well, she says she knows you. And she knew you last year and y'all were together. She was only 17 last year and now she's 18."

Horace was basically accusing me of statutory rape. (Ed. note: *Legal age for consensual sex in the state of Utah is 18.*) "I swear to you, I don't know this chick."

Mark jumped in at that point. "Brian says he doesn't know her. You said you don't know her, right, Brian?"

"That's exactly what I'm saying."

"The father says different," Horace said.

"Well, let's get him on the phone, too," Mark said.

Game 2 is several hours away and now I'm on a conference call with my agent, NBA head of security, and the dad of a teenage daughter. "My daughter says she met you at the mall," the father said. "You take advantage of young girls. You take advantage of little girls."

"I don't know your fucking daughter!"

Then we heard a female voice in the background say, "Hey, Dad," and he responded, "Oh, hey, honey."

He started up again about how I had taken advantage of his daughter when we heard, "Dad, what are you doing?"

"I'm telling them about Brian Grant," the dad says.

"Dad, I fucking told you I don't know that guy. He was *with* the guy at the mall that I was with. He doesn't know me! Why would you?"

"Oh," the dad says. "I thought you said he knew you."

Mark cussed the dad out. When the dad hung up, all he said was, "Alright, goodbye."

Horace got it from Mark next. After we hung up with him, I was still shook. I've got to face Karl Malone and the Jazz in a playoff game in a couple of hours and I'm sitting there thinking, 'Did I sleep with somebody and not remember?" I never went anywhere other than the mall in Salt Lake City, but when you get accused of something that serious it makes you think.

And maybe that was the real purpose behind the whole accusation. It felt like the dad knew it would have me mentally distracted for the game, regardless of it being true or not. That might sound far-fetched, but not to anybody who knows Utah Jazz fans. I don't know how, but there were people at the game who knew all about the accusation, too. One guy in the stands said to me, "You like little girls, Brian? Was she good?" Another guy started shouting the girl's name while I was shooting a free throw. There was even a guy in the seats behind one of the backboards with a sign that read, "You like minors, Brian?"

The guy in Washington (Ed. note: *Notorious heckler Robin Ficker, a Washington Bullets fan who had season tickets behind the visiting team bench*) was really tough, too, but he did his homework. He'd know everything about you and hit you with these wicked jabs. "How's the family life, Brian?" Guys would be begging to get back in the game so they wouldn't have to listen to him.

But I want to thank that dad and those Jazz fans because they lit a fire under my ass. Once the ball went up, I was motivated, not distracted. I played Karl almost even and the referees actually treated us as equals. He dominated the boards with 17 rebounds, but we both scored 23 points—including nine each from free throws. JR was the biggest difference maker for us, making four of six three-pointers for 27 points. All of that was enough for an 84–81 win, sending us to Portland with the series tied 1–1.

Our depth and Utah's age really showed themselves the next two games in front of our fans at the Rose Garden. It worked in our favor that they were on back-to-back nights. In Game 3, we had six players score in double figures; they had three. We led by six at the end of the first quarter and never trailed again, winning 97–87.

Game 4 may have been the surest sign that the Jazz tread was finally wearing thin after more than a decade of running over people. It was the kind of ugly, grinding game they were famous for winning—and they didn't. Sabas (15 rebounds, 14 points) and JR (24 points, including 10 free throws) had a lot to do with that. This time we made the fourth-quarter comeback, outscoring them 25–17 for an 81–75 win. Both Karl (17 points, 11 rebounds) and John (16 points, 10 assists) had double-doubles, but we won the battle around the basket as a team. Of our 25 points in the fourth quarter, 22 were from free throws or shots in the paint.

Karl even threw me a compliment after Game 4, telling reporters that I'd done "a great job in the series so far." When they relayed that back to me, I told them it was "an honor" to play against him. I meant it. But all the flowery talk about each other evaporated pretty quickly in Game 5.

The Jazz were fighting for their playoff lives, so we knew they were capable of doing almost anything, especially in their own building. Near the end of the first quarter, Karl and I went up for a rebound. He mistimed his jump and went up too early. I had just started to jump as he was coming down, his elbows out. One caught me between my eye and my forehead, the full weight of Karl's 250 pounds behind it. I saw a lightning flash and my vision blurred. I nearly fell over but managed to get my hands down to keep myself from hitting the floor. When I stood up, blood was streaming down my face. There was no concussion protocol the way there is today, so the only thing that could keep me from continuing to play was if we couldn't stop the bleeding. They walked me back to the locker room, sewed up the gash with six stitches, slapped a couple of band-aids over it, and I was good to go.

There's something about playing in the Delta Center when Karl and John seem to be getting every whistle from the refs and the crowd is roaring and talking shit that can get under your skin. The first row of seats are almost directly behind the visiting bench, which makes it feel as if their fans are right in your ear the whole night, and they take full advantage of being that close. We also had a reputation as a team for being a little wild, and it always seemed as if the refs were expecting trouble from us.

The Jazz led by 10 after the first quarter and we couldn't make enough shots to slow them down. What put all of us over the edge was the feeling that it wasn't a fair fight. Karl didn't get a technical or a foul for hitting me with that elbow. But when I grabbed a rebound early in the fourth quarter, I was immediately hit with a technical foul for swinging my elbows, even though I didn't make contact with anything but the air. Less than a minute later, I grabbed another rebound, and this time, Karl leaned in and smacked me right on the funny bone in my elbow. I swear it's a trick of his because he got me more than once like that. My elbow burned and went numb for a second.

I've taken an elbow to the face with no call, I've been T'ed up while not touching anyone, we're getting our asses kicked, and now Karl is whacking my elbow and getting away with it?

For a split second, I lost my cool and faked as if I was going to throw the ball at him. I didn't actually throw it and Karl had already started running back down the court so he didn't even see it, but the way things were going, when I heard a whistle I thought I had been hit with another technical, so I just walked to the other end of the court before I completely lost my cool. It turned out Mike saw Karl's whack on my elbow and had walked onto the court to yell at referee Ron Garretson for letting him get away with it, prompting Garretson to T up Mike, not me.

The technical foul, though, only made Mike more mad and he had to be held back by our assistant coaches and a couple of our players. That earned him a second technical from Garretson and an automatic ejection.

Karl was headed to his bench when I decided to let him know that he could throw all the elbows and cheap shots he wanted, but that I wasn't going to back down. Those weren't my exact words—the exact words started with an "f" and a "b" and maybe an "m." We were nose to nose but I wasn't going to touch him because then I knew it would have been on. He was as calm as a placid lake the whole time.

As soon as the game was over, I walked into the locker room, grabbed my clothes, stuffed them in my bag, and got on the team bus still funky and sweaty because I didn't want to talk to anybody. I was still pissed off. Everybody else eventually got on the bus, and as they passed my seat, patted me and said, "Alright, big fella, way to go."

The bus took us to the airport that night to fly home, with Game 6 in Portland. Gina was still up when I walked through the door. "How's your eye?" she asked.

"It's good," I said. "I'm alright."

"Elijah was crying his eyes out," she said of our one-year-old son. "He kept saying, 'He hurt my daddy!'"

"I'll tell him I'm alright in the morning."

"Did you hear what Karl Malone said?"

"No. I went straight to the bus after the game. I haven't heard or seen anything. What did he say?"

It was starting to get light out. We turned on ESPN's *SportsCenter* and sat back on the couch. There he was in front of the cameras and microphones. "I don't like him and he don't like me," he told the reporters. "I'm not here to make friends and I don't give a damn that I elbowed him in the eye. It's gonna be an all-out war. We're here to win a game. And whatever it takes to win, that's how we gonna do. We're gonna win."

I watched the clip of Karl more than once, taking it all in and getting myself ready for what was to come, because I knew several things were going to happen as a result of Karl saying all that. One, the media was going to be all over me looking for a response. Two, the referees were going to go into the game concerned something might jump off between us and, as I knew all too well, they were more likely to come down on me than Karl if anything got started.

Sure enough, the media were set up and waiting for me the next day and didn't waste time getting to what everyone wanted to know. "Okay, Brian," someone started. "Karl Malone had some choice words for you last night. He says he's not your friend and he's not here to make friends. What do you have to say to Karl?"

For someone who was afraid of getting drafted because it would mean having to go up on stage and say a few words of thanks, I wasn't the least bit nervous. I'd like to think I was as calm as Karl was when I was in his face telling him what I thought of his elbows and his cheap shots.

"Well, first of all, he's my idol," I said. "He's the one that I patterned my game off of, you know? I heard he likes to go fishing and I'm hoping that one day we can go fishing together."

Someone asked about the elbow and I simply said, "That's all I gotta say." A couple of the reporters groaned. I'm sure they had been hoping I would go back at Karl. But I left feeling glad I hadn't talked to anybody right after the game because I certainly wouldn't have come up with the kill-'em-with-kindness approach then.

The people of Portland let me know how they felt about me the next night. As we waited in the tunnel to get our cue to run onto the court to warm up, you could already hear the crowd roaring and it had all of us revved up. When we finally ran out of the tunnel and into the bowl of the arena, it was so loud it felt like you had to push the sound out of the way to get to the court. When I looked up into the stands, everyone was cheering and pointing to their foreheads. Every one of them—fans, ushers, vendors—had a band-aid over their right eye. I'd never seen a show of solidarity like that, for anything, ever. Everybody was so hyped up it was almost scary.

But all of that put me in a zone. I knew what everybody in that arena expected me to do and I wasn't about to let them down. I told Mike, "When he goes in, I go in. When he goes out, I go out. I'll stay out of foul trouble. And even if it looks like I'm getting in foul trouble, I won't put myself in a position where I can pick up any more."

I didn't have to say who "he" was.

If Mike trusted somebody, he'd roll with them every chance he could. Mike trusted I'd do what I said or die trying. "Alright," Mike said. "He's yours."

I made it through the first quarter without a single foul and Mike stuck to his word, actually keeping me on the floor 10 seconds longer than Karl. I'd like to think diffusing the war of words, at least from my end, had something to do with the referees treating me fairly. I picked up two fouls in the second quarter, though, and Mike sat me for almost three minutes while Karl played the entire period; some of that might've been punishment for wasting a foul on Thurl Bailey. In the third quarter, though, Karl played 11 minutes and 45 seconds—and so did I, while picking up only one more foul.

More important than all that though, was Karl couldn't find the basket. At halftime he had three points on six shots and one rebound. He tried to get going in the third quarter, taking eight shots, but he only made two.

The fourth quarter was actually worse—he went scoreless on two shots. It was a very un-Karl Malone performance: 3-for-16 for eight points and seven rebounds. He only outscored me by one and I had 12 rebounds. With JR and Jim Jackson combining to go a perfect 22-for-22 from the free-throw line, we pulled away in the fourth quarter for a 92–80 win.

Every ounce of my energy had gone into making the game hard for Karl. With the confetti falling from the rafters and my teammates celebrating and the fans still screaming, he found me on the court afterward. "Brian, you know I didn't mean any of that," he said. "Man, I think you're a hell of a player. Good luck. Keep playing hard."

"Thank you," I said. I told him everything I'd told reporters before the game—that I looked up to him and had patterned my game after him—*was* true. That's why no trophy or award could've ever meant more than Karl telling me I'd done a good job against him. I really didn't even care what anybody said or thought about my performance after that. Not that I didn't pay a price. My knees ached, especially my left one, and my whole body felt as banged up as that spot just above my right eye. Nor was there time to soak in Karl's respect, because I had an even tougher assignment waiting for me in facing the top-seeded San Antonio Spurs and their All-Star power forward, Tim Duncan.

As a team, though, we were not thinking about the Spurs. We had to fight through so many incidents and expend so much emotion in beating the Jazz, it felt like the Finals, and we celebrated like it. Looking back, we probably did too much celebrating. These were not the Spurs you think of now—a dynasty that lasted well over a decade and won five championships. They were trying to break through for the first time just like we were. But that's probably what made them more dangerous; they had just swept the Kobe-Shaq Lakers on their side of the bracket and they shook hands with each other and walked off the floor as if it were just another game.

For me, facing Tim was completely different than dealing with Malone. It was all about scrapping with Karl. He had quickness and strength and loved to drive into you. Since I always felt like I was behind the eight-ball with the refs I had to be careful how I dealt with that, but defensively I had more success against Karl than with Tim. Long players with post games gave me the most trouble, and that's exactly what Tim was.

Karl got a lot of his buckets by beating every other big man down the floor for layups off Stockton-led fastbreaks and mid-range jumpers. He was 35 and this had been his 14th season. Tim, on the other hand, was practically fresh out of the box—22 years old and finishing up his second season. He could run the floor, too, but not like Karl. He had a jumper, too, but not like Karl's. He didn't blaze past you as much as he tricked you. At 6'11" he was taller than Karl by a couple of inches and he had long-ass arms on top of that. If he got to his turnaround with either hand, it was money every time. But if you went to block the turnaround, he'd hit you with an up-and-under. He didn't have a great vertical jump, but he was so long he'd make you change your shot. His hands sucked in the ball if it was anywhere near him and never seemed to lose it.

What wasn't different between Karl and Tim is how often both of their teams used them offensively—which was pretty much every time down the floor. After wrestling with Karl for six games in 10 days, I had 48 hours to get ready to face Tim in the Alamodome.

This may sound like I'm trying to discount what the Spurs did to us, but it didn't feel like we lost four straight games to them, even though we did. The first game was so ugly I don't even remember most of the details. Neither team played well, but we were only down by two points with a minute and 40 seconds left. The problem was, we were down by the same two points, 78–76, with four seconds left. The Spurs deserve a lot of credit for that. They were arguably the best defensive team in the league, with two future Hall of Famers in Duncan and center David Robinson protecting the rim and Gregg Popovich as their head coach.

It looked as if we were ready to do what we had done against the Jazz—take a disappointing loss in Game 1 and then make up for it with a dominating performance in Game 2. We led by 11 after the first quarter and had a 52–34 lead early in the third quarter. Our bench had a lot to do with that, outscoring their subs 27–6 for the game, but that's because we had to lean on them more than usual. Neither Arvydas nor JR played a minute in the fourth quarter because they had some physical issues. The Spurs took advantage, steadily closing the gap.

But we never lost the lead and it was still our game to win when Damon made a free throw with 12 seconds left to put us up 85–83. Up to this point, the Spurs were a lot like us—a talented team with lots of potential but always falling one play or one basket short of getting over the hump. If you made a run on them, especially late in the game, you could feel their fans getting nervous. It almost made up for playing in the Dome, which was built as a football stadium in hopes of luring a pro team there. The depth perception was off with all that empty space behind the backboards, making it hard to judge how far you were from the basket.

Sean Elliott did not seem to have a problem with it in Game 2, resulting in what is known as "The Memorial Day Miracle" ever since. Mario Elie inbounded the ball straight down the right sideline with a pass that looked like it might either get intercepted or sail out of bounds. Stacey Augmon went for the steal but the ball flew just past his fingertips. His man, Elliott, caught it but went up on his toes to do so and looked as if he were about to fall out of bounds as he grabbed the ball.

That's when it got really crazy.

Now, Sean was a big reason the Spurs made it back from being so far behind. He singlehandedly cut our 18-point lead in half with three three-pointers. But as I remember, they were all shots where they swung the ball to him, he caught it, and hit an open shot.

This time he caught the ball with his back to the basket, pivoted—still on his tip-toes—took one dribble to his right, and launched a shot. If you go back and watch, his heels are over the out-of-bounds line almost the entire time. If he puts them down, as anyone would naturally do to catch their balance before shooting, he's out of bounds, it's our ball, and the game is over.

But he doesn't. He never put his heels down. Instead, he shot the ball.

I couldn't see him let go of it because Sheed, recognizing that Stacey went for the steal and didn't get it, ran out at Sean, leaped, and stretched as high as he could. And again, the same way Elie's pass just slipped past Stacey's fingertips, Sean's shot just scraped past Sheed's.

And then found nothing but net. The Alamodome fans lost their minds. The Spurs celebrated the way we did after beating the Jazz. And we walked to the locker room, every one of us with a what-just-happened look on our face.

It's hard to admit, but we weren't just stunned. We were devastated. That loss let the proverbial air out of our tires.

The Spurs sensed it, too. We went back to Portland and they blasted us, twice, on our home floor, to close the series, 4–0. That put them where we wanted to be, the Finals, with a bonus—they would face the eighth-seeded New York Knicks, who started the playoffs by upsetting the No. 1 seed Miami Heat and took out the second-seeded Indiana Pacers in the Eastern Conference finals. The Knicks were built around Latrell Sprewell and Allan Houston, perimeter players, and had no way of slowing down Tim and David. It took San Antonio five games to win four and claim the title.

I'd like to think they would've had just as much trouble with our front line and that could've been the start of a dynasty in Portland. If winning a championship is like climbing Mt. Everest, we weren't quite at the peak, but we celebrated like we were—and wound up never making it up those last few feet. Which meant I got to witness, up close, the turning point that changed a close-but-no-cigar team into a champion.

Not for the last time, either.

chapter 8

Odd Man Out

Although making it to the Western Conference finals ended a stretch of six consecutive first-round exits by the Blazers, we all knew our GM, Bob Whitsitt, would not be satisfied and changes were coming. Sure enough, JR and Jim Jackson were traded to the Atlanta Hawks for Ed Gray and Steve Smith. But "Trader Bob," as he was known, wasn't done. Right before training camp started he sent practically half our team—Augmon, Kelvin Cato, Gray, Carlos Rogers, Brian Shaw, and Walt Williams—to the Houston Rockets for Scottie Pippen.

It wasn't hard to figure out what he had in mind: he wanted our team to grow up—fast.

I looked at us as a band of misfits all thrown together. And not because of anything having to do with us being called the Jail Blazers—I didn't even find out someone had tagged us that until much later. It was one of those teams where if somebody was acting out of pocket, it was on them. If you're a misfit, it feels hypocritical to call somebody out for being a misfit. I remember after one practice seeing JR being interviewed and I decided to walk by and eavesdrop on what he was saying. I walked up just in time to hear a reporter ask him if he thought there was racism in Oregon. "You can probably go 20 miles down the road and they're still lynching brothers," JR said.

"Damn," I thought, chuckling to myself. I slipped away before anyone asked me to comment on JR's comment. Did anybody say anything to him about that comment? Not any of the players. The way we saw it, whatever anybody was doing that might be out of line, that was on Mike to clean it up. JR had a habit of being late for practice and Mike was hoping we'd handle it. When we didn't, he started making us all wait to get started until JR showed up. I guess that was supposed to make us mad at JR or get us to say something to him, but it didn't work. We just weren't like that with each other.

You've probably heard and read a lot of negative comments about JR, but I'm not about to add to them. He's one of the most talented cats I've ever played with or against. Athletically, he could jump out of the gym. He could shoot, go hard to the basket, and defend when he wanted to. If we needed a bucket, that's who we looked to first. He was a good teammate 99.9 percent of the time. I know when he lost his mother it was hard on him for a long while and he struggled, so I was happy to hear that he was working with kids and seemed to have found his way back.

JR walked to his own beat—but we all did, in a way. You had me, dreaded out and pure energy at power forward. You had a 7-footer in Sabonis, who looked like a typical big ol' slow center but had the passing and long-range-shooting skills of a point guard long before that became fashionable with big men. There was Sheed, who would dunk on anybody any chance he had and then added a three-point shot as well. And Damon, one of the first undersized scoring point guards. We had so many pieces and egos, you couldn't call it "a team." That's why I called us a band of misfits.

For anybody who wonders why NBA players sometimes do what they do, it's because you feel like you're living in a fairy tale and you think it's going to last forever. You're not thinking 10 years down the road. You're in your twenties and making more money and have more toys than you ever dreamed of. You look around and you're not alone, either. The majority of the cats around you are living the same way, walking to their own beat. So why would you do anything different? Because someone who is not in the NBA thinks you should? Someone whose life is nothing like yours?

Bob understood that, which is why he brought in 30-year-old Steve and 34-year-old Scottie and signed 36-year-old free agent Detlef Schrempf, who Bob had traded for six years earlier when he was the Sonics' GM. He also brought back 31-year-old Stacey after the Rockets waived him.

Bob wanted them to influence the younger crowd on our team—me, Sheed, Jermaine, Bonzi Wells, and Damon. He was hoping their professionalism would rub off on us.

We called them The Suits. They called us The Sweatsuits.

We were all cool with each other, but on the bus and the plane we had our separate sections—and on the team plane Paul Allen provided, we were really separate. Paul's wealth and what he provided his teams (he owned the Seattle Seahawks as well) was something I had to get used to after being in Sacramento. It's not as if the Kings' owners were cheap; they just weren't loaded the way Paul was. The Blazers' team plane looked more like a spaceship. The Suits sat closer to the front and played poker. The Sweatsuits sat in the back with headphones listening to music or watching movies.

I could hang with either group. I'd be up with The Suits— Greg Anthony was with them, too—and they'd ask, "What are they doing back there?" I'd go back to find out and someone would ask, "What are those busters up there talking about?" And then someone would throw in a shot, like, "Man, go tell Scottie them damn shoes don't look right." That might start a smack-talk exchange and I'd be the messenger. On some teams you might worry about cliques creating divisions in the team that eventually show up on the court, but it wasn't like that. We accepted our differences. It was fun.

Being part of both groups helped me get over the fact that I'd lost my starting job. Having to deal with Karl and Tim had worn down the cartilage in my left knee, requiring microfracture surgery. Technically, they called it "a lateral release with a microfracture repair." Some of my deepest conversations were with doctors and team trainers; I wanted to understand what it was they were doing to my body. My left knee apparently tracked out, so they cut tissue on the outside and shaved the area on the inside to eliminate a divot that had developed. And then they drilled holes into the bone to let the bone marrow bleed out and toughen into a layer to replace the cartilage buffer in your knee. Sounds heavy, right? They might've discouraged me at Xavier from getting a degree in medicine, but I swear I earned at least a few credits learning all I did about my injuries and surgeries.

The standard protocol after microfracture is that you not put weight on it for six to eight weeks. At the start, they strap your leg into a perpetual motion machine for six hours a day. It's supposed to take four to six months before you can return to any sort of sports activity, six to eight months to return to amateur competition, and it can take a year before the knee is ready to endure the physical stress of being a pro.

You can guess how well I followed all that. Between believing I could get my body to do whatever my mind asked of it and wanting to be on a basketball court every minute I could, I was back working out in 4½ months; a few weeks after that I played my first game.

I spent the first two weeks of the regular season on the inactive list, getting back into shape in practice. Sheed moved back into the starting power forward spot and Scottie became the starting small forward. I wasn't mad about it—he could've made a fuss when I first came to Portland and Dunleavy moved him to small forward, but he rolled with it. Besides, I knew how good Sheed was. A lot of guys say it, but I truly mean it—I wanted to win more than I wanted personal accolades. Respect the work I'm putting in, show that you want the best for me, and we're cool.

I also knew Mike had his hands full. I knew the first day of the first year that he was going to have a hard time, not just keeping everybody happy but not having somebody go off and do or say something crazy. You have guys on every team who think they should be playing more or getting more shots, but on the Blazers the frustration level was higher because it was true. Detlef and me had been starters and Jermaine and Bonzi were young but certainly talented enough to start. It made our practices as exciting as our games, but it put pressure on everybody. One bad practice and you might see your minutes slip. The starters had to fight to keep their spots and the subs had to fight to keep their roles. Our guys all had big personalities, too, which meant they weren't going to be shy about letting everybody know how they felt about anything that bothered them. Mike did the best he could, but it was a circus.

Even though we won 13 of our first 15 games, Mike considered moving me back into the starting lineup once I got back into shape. I was okay with whatever he wanted to do, but I didn't think it was the right move. I didn't want to rock the boat and Sheed was ballin'. It never came down to him asking and me saying no; I just know he thought about it at one point. It wasn't as simple as just starting the best five. He had to figure out how to get the most out of everybody without having us step on each other's toes. With only one ball, he needed guys who could impact the game without it. I could do that with my defense and rebounding. It worked out. Sheed wound up making the Western Conference All-Star team and we barely slowed down the rest of the way, finishing 59–23.

No matter how many games we won, though, we knew there was only one accomplishment that would satisfy Whitsitt: a championship. Paul probably felt that way, too, since we had the most expensive team in the league, something that wouldn't happen in a small market like Portland without a billionaire owner who never pinched pennies with either the Blazers or the

Seahawks. Bob clearly had Paul's blessing to keep reshuffling the team's deck of players in search of a championship combination.

Not that any of us had a problem with that thinking. We had the same feeling.

The idea of me going back to the starting lineup ended when I missed nearly another month of action with plantar fasciitis in my left foot. I'd been dealing with it all year, but the bottom of my foot finally got so swollen I could barely walk on it. There's no cure for it other than ice and rest. In a way it's worse than having torn cartilage or a torn labrum because they can surgically fix those and you know how long you're supposed to be out. With plantar fasciitis you have just to wait until it stops feeling like you're stepping on hot needles. Pain was something I learned to play through, but it can get to the point where you just can't do your job and you're hurting the team.

With everything about the season feeling do-or-die, I was as fired up for the playoffs as I would've been starting. After the shot Sean Elliott pulled out of his... imagination, I had it hard-wired into my brain that an entire series can flip on one play or possession. If there was a play like that this time around, I sure as hell wanted to do everything I could to be on the side celebrating.

Remember I told you that.

I know as well as anyone what it's like to take the court with life off the court throwing curveballs. Our entire team was going through that as we faced our first-round opponent, the Minnesota Timberwolves and their All-Star power forward, Kevin Garnett. One of our assistant coaches, Bill Musselman, was at the Mayo Clinic in Rochester, Minnesota, being treated for bone cancer.

It had been a rough year for Bill and a sad one for all of us. He was an old dude, 59, and had suffered a stroke during training camp. That's when they first discovered the cancer as well. If you didn't know him, you might take one look and think he was just one of those old heads a team keeps around as a calming influence, but Bill knew his stuff.

We couldn't blame our habit of losing focus on Bill's condition. As soon as we put ourselves in the driver's seat, we'd get lazy or start looking ahead, forgetting that any team good enough to be in the playoffs was too good to take for granted—especially a team that had KG. Even though Sheed was a tough matchup for him and we had several guys who could take turns guarding KG, he never stopped battling. If you came half-stepping, he was going to bust your ass all night. It was almost as if he took it as an insult that you weren't playing your hardest against him.

I don't know how deep the Timberwolves' pride ran, but I know how deep it ran with KG. He had to know he was out-manned facing us, but he wasn't about to accept being swept out of a series, on his home floor, no less. Our tendency to fall into thinking our talent alone could carry us, combined with KG going off for his second triple-double of the series, cost us Game 3.

Before Game 4, "Muss" called each one of us with a few words of advice and encouragement. His surgery was scheduled for the next day. He left a message on my phone, telling me I was a hell of a player and to keep working because I had a bright future. At the end of the message he said, "It was an honor to coach you." He was crying.

We all decided to dedicate Game 4 to him. I'd like to tell you that inspired us to crush the Timberwolves from start to finish; actually, we struggled for the first three quarters. Our depth and versatility came through for us in the end. KG finished one assist short of a third triple-double, but it didn't matter. We were on fire, outscoring Minnesota 28–13 in the fourth quarter. We all signed the game ball and had it sent to Muss to see when he came out of surgery. It wasn't enough. A couple days after the operation and on the eve of our first second-round game, we got word that Muss had passed. We had a funeral service just for people with the Blazers and his son, Eric. When Mike talked to the media right before the next series started, he could barely speak.

As a team, Bill's death could've hit us one of two ways—distracted us or motivated us.

But we were already pretty dialed in to take care of business against the Jazz. In one way, we had already proven that Whitsitt's off-season moves had made us better. But how much better? Better enough to win a championship? Because that's all that mattered. And the Jazz would give us a way to measure all that.

We also had a weapon that we hadn't had the year before—a guy who *expected* to beat the Jazz any time he faced them. If there was anyone who was not going to be intimidated in the series, it was Scottie. Plenty of players hated playing against the Jazz, especially in the Delta Center, for good reason. Not a lot of teams went in there and had success. John and Karl knew how to work the refs and the fans—well, you know how the fans can be from what I told you about what happened the last time I was in Salt Lake City for the playoffs.

Whatever the fans might say to Scottie, all he had to do was raise two fingers—not as a peace sign but as a reminder of the number of championships he'd won by beating the Jazz when he was with the Bulls. With Michael retired, Scottie might've been the one player who could walk into the Delta Center and make the *home* team uncomfortable.

Since we had the better record, the series started with the first two games in the Rose Garden. Whether it was that, our squad being better, or Karl and John being a year older, we made Whitsitt look smart in the first two games, blowing out the Jazz in both. It probably had a lot to do with Scottie, who was a much tougher matchup at both ends for the Jazz's third star, Hornacek. We exploited that. JR had always been focused on scoring, but now we had Smitty (Steve Smith) for that. Scottie, meanwhile, loved nothing more than to shut somebody down, which is why he had been named to the league's All-Defensive team for an ninth year in a row.

Game 3 was more of the same, giving us a chance to sweep. We couldn't help but see ourselves as unstoppable. Beating the Jazz is a huge confidence boost for any team, but smashing them three times and possibly sweeping them? Even when the Bulls beat them in the Finals, it took them six games both times.

It wasn't hard for me to imagine what the Jazz were feeling—we had been in this same position just a year earlier. No NBA team has ever come back to win a seven-game playoff series from a 3–0 hole and this may come as a shock to fans, but teams don't just quit. If you're up against a playoff team and aren't all in on trying to win, you're not only going to lose, you're going to get embarrassed—and any team good enough to make the playoffs is too proud to just let that happen.

I never had a problem finding motivation, in part because I always had something to prove to someone. If you didn't think I could get the job done, I had to prove I could. If you thought I could get the job done, then I had to prove you were right. I also had a lifetime of firsthand experiences that showed no matter who you were, no matter where you came from, you could rise to the top or get squashed to the bottom.

Which is why I came off the bench and played my ass off against Karl—20 points and 13 rebounds in 26 minutes. After Karl showed me all that respect after last year's series, the best way I could thank him was by playing him tough all over again.

Despite all that, we couldn't quite put them away. Karl had a great game, too—27 points, eight rebounds, seven assists. We weren't feeling ourselves quite the same way after the 88–85 loss, but we were going home and still led the series 3–1.

Thank God Bryon Russell is not Sean Elliott. Game 5 came down to the wire the same as Game 4, where we had a chance to send it to overtime but missed a three-pointer at the buzzer. Just as in Game 2 with the Spurs, we were holding a two-point lead, this time with 1.4 seconds left. The Jazz got the ball to Bryon Russell, who got off his shot with—guess who—Sheed running to block it. This time there was no miracle. We were headed back to the Western Conference finals to face the only team with a better regular-season record, the team who thought *they* were the next dynasty. It was also a team that had lit my fire since the start of my NBA career.

These were not the same Lakers I'd faced my first year in Portland. They were *way* better. Kobe had broken out of his shell and taken his first steps to becoming the Mamba, Shaq had been named league MVP, and Phil Jackson had replaced Del Harris as head coach. If there was any team that could match us in egos and confidence, it was the Lakers.

As good as Kobe was, figuring out what to do with Shaq was our biggest challenge. On paper, we looked to have the answer in Sabonis, who came as close to matching Shaq in size and strength as anyone in the league. But Shaq had taken his handle and spin moves to another level. Not only was Sabonis struggling to stop him, he was getting into foul trouble trying, and that meant we didn't have his passing and scoring on offense.

Game 1 was a perfect example. Shaq damn near played the whole game like a league MVP—41 points, 11 rebounds, seven assists, and five blocked shots. We could usually count on Sabas to come through for us in big games but he went scoreless and only grabbed one rebound in 33 minutes. Sheed got tossed for looking at referee Ron Garretson a certain way in the third quarter. Granted, Sheed had some hardcore looks, but it was better than saying, "Fucking cheater." Which is what Sheed might say to a ref if he thought it was warranted. Bottom line, the Lakers won easily, 109–94.

We were feeling pretty discouraged in the locker room until Scottie came in and gave a really good speech about how our mission was simply to win one in L.A. and we still had a chance to do that if we came correct in Game 2. That clicked with us.

Mike knew by now I enjoyed taking on bigger, better players. Taking on Shaq, though, would certainly be the biggest and the best. I would be giving up at least 75 pounds in weight and four inches in height—and that was just the physical part. He wasn't the Shaq in Orlando who could run the floor and dunk lobs on your ass; I'm glad when I was in Sacramento that job went to Duane Causwell, because I couldn't have done anything with that Shaq. He'd gotten bigger and stronger, learned how to get you to lean on him and then spin off you for a little baby jump hook with either hand. Phil did a good job of getting him the ball while he was on the move, making it even harder to keep him from running you over and drawing a blocking foul on you. Mike hoped my quickness and willingness to give up my body might, if nothing else, keep Sabas out of foul trouble and making plays on offense.

"You think you can handle Shaq?" Mike asked.

"Hell, yeah," I said. I'd been David my whole career. This was a chance to take on the biggest Goliath in the game.

I also had a plan that, if it worked, would make Shaq have to think about me a little bit, too.

The first trick to guarding Shaq was knowing when you should try. The first few minutes of a game? Forget it. A man that big and fast, when he's fresh and frothing at the mouth, there's no stopping that. You just have to let him be Shaq. The only thing I'd do early is get into his body and pound his ribs with my forearm a few times, whether he had the ball or not. That might make him mad and he'd spin past me for a dunk, but once he made that drop-step I'd let him go. As soon as the ball went through the hoop, though, I'd grab it, inbound it and sprint down the court. Even if he wasn't guarding me, it meant he had to bust it back on D or we'd be playing five-on-four. I did everything I could do to force him to keep moving. I think if you asked him, he'd say he respected how hard I worked.

Once he was winded, I had a chance to stay between him and the basket and make him shoot over me. He didn't have quite the same balance or accuracy when he was a little gassed.

I wouldn't want to say that's why we blew out the Lakers in Game 2, 106–77, but it played a part. Shaq had 23 points, a solid game for anybody else, but below his standard. The Lakers might've been feeling themselves a little bit after the first game, too. It also helped that the refs and Sheed left each other alone. Mike must've figured he was well-rested after not getting to play the fourth quarter in Game 1, so he played Sheed 46 of the 48 minutes, even though it was a blowout.

Looking back, I don't think I've ever seen or been part of a series with so many gut checks. We were like two big dudes in a bar, throwing haymakers. Just when you thought one of us was staggered and about to fall, that team would turn around and connect with a solid shot that had the other team wobbling.

The Lakers got the next two punches in, both on our home floor. We lost Game 3 by two points, 93–91, and maybe that

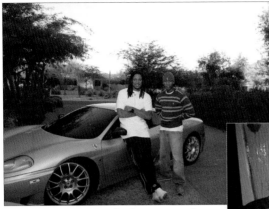

Phoenix, Arizona, in the driveway with great friend Raphael Saadiq.

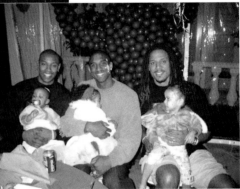

Me with Kobe Bryant (center) and Caron Butler (left) at Kobe's daughter Natalia's birthday party in 2005.

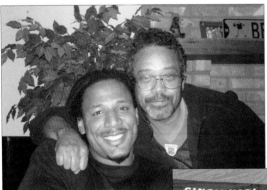

Me and my dad watching a Bengals game in 2006.

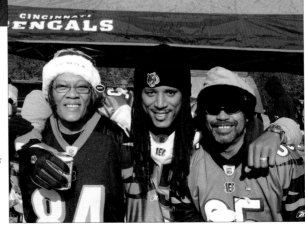

Cincinnati Bengals game, 2006, with Mom and Dad.

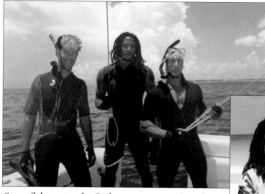

Spearfishing in the Bahamas in 2006 with Phillipe Manicom (left) and Dodd Romero (right).

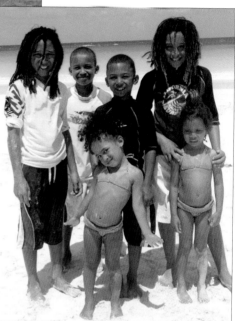

Our 2006 family trip to the Bahamas: Elijah (left), Jonavan (middle left), Anaya (bottom), Jaydon (middle right), Amani (top right), and Maliah (bottom right).

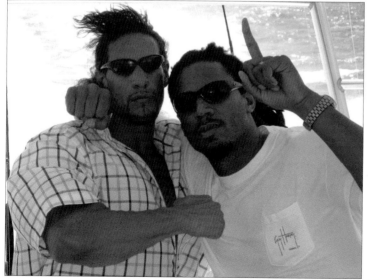

My friend and trainer, Dodd Romero (left), and me on my boat in 2007, as we made our way to the Bahamas from Miami.

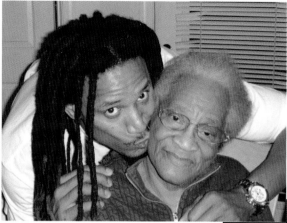

Me with my Mamaw Lizzy at a 2007 family reunion.

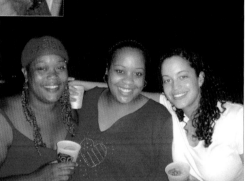

My younger sisters at a family reunion (from left): Brianna, Stephanie, and Lakisha.

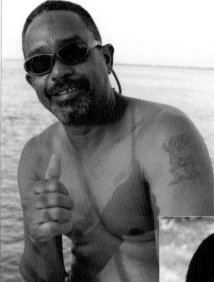

My dad on a fishing trip with me.

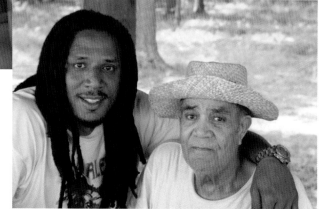

And me and Papaw (Elwood) Grant at a family reunion.

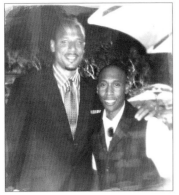

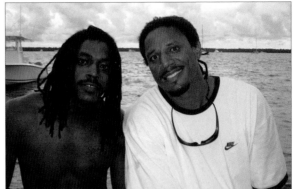

Me and my great friend Raphael Saadiq at Holly Robinson-Peete's 2007 fundraising gala.

Boat day in Miami, 2007: my younger brother, Brandon (left), and me.

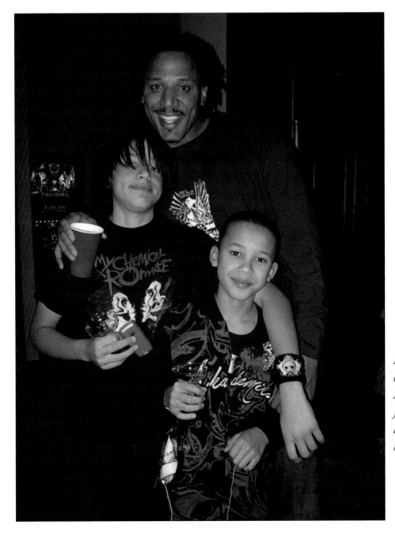

Me with two of my sons, Amani (left) and Jonavan (right), at my Oregon home in 2008.

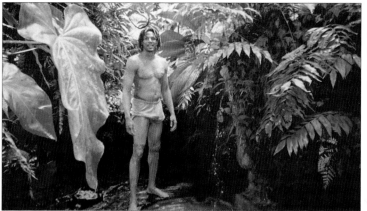

Here I am in a jungle in Dominica after mud healing.

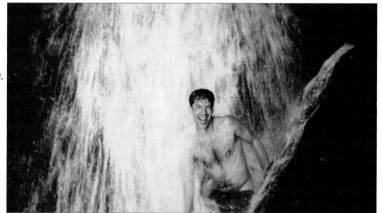

Phillipe Manicom under a waterfall on a trip to Dominica.

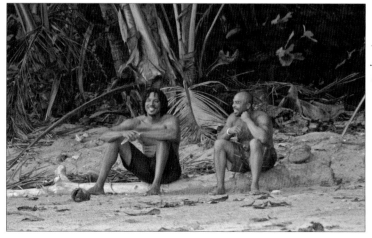

Me and my cousin Jermaine Marshall in Costa Rica.

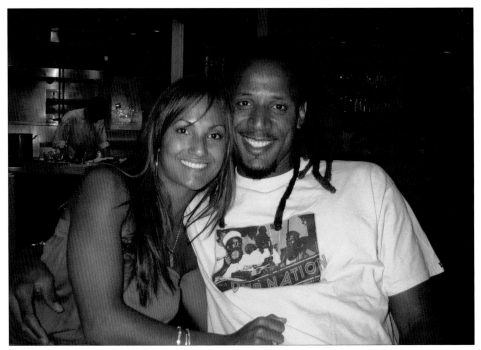

Me and Gina at dinner in Cannes, France.

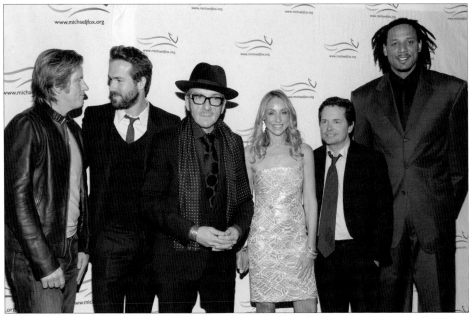

From left: Denis Leary, Ryan Reynolds, Elvis Costello, Tracy Pollan, Michael J. Fox, and me at the A Funny Thing Happened on the Way to Cure Parkinson's benefit in New York in November 2009. (AP Images/Evan Agostini)

Here I am holding my Xavier jersey at the number retirement ceremony, which took place at halftime of a game between Xavier and Temple.
(AP Images/Al Behrman)

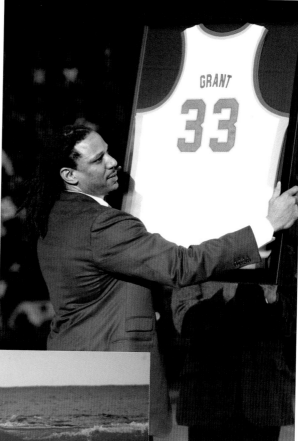

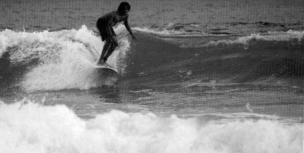

Me in Costa Rica catching a wave.

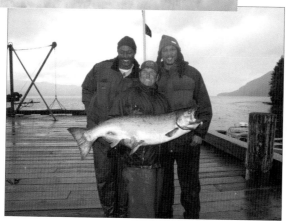

Karl Malone (left) and me stand with our guide on our Alaskan fishing trip that was auctioned off at the Shake It Till We Make It gala in 2013.

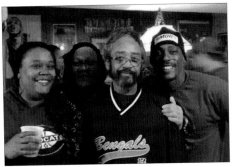

Family get together, 2016 (from left): Brianna, Mom, Dad, and Brandon.

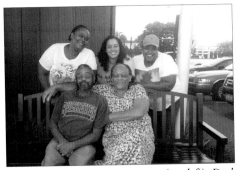

My parents and sisters: Brianna (top left), Dad (bottom left), Lakisha (top middle), Mom (bottom right), and Stephanie (top right).

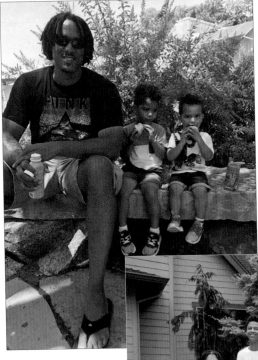

Hanging at the zoo in Madison, Wisconsin, with my two youngest sons, Brian (middle) and Maxwell (right).

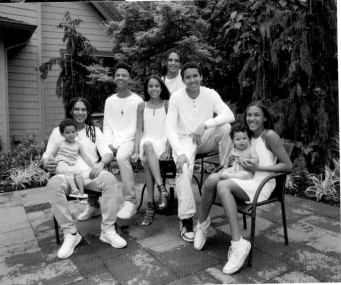

My kids at my Oregon home in 2016 (from left): Brian, Elijah, Jaydon, Maliah, Amani, Jonavan, Maxwell, and Anaya.

had us thinking we just needed to do one or two things better and we'd get Game 4. Nope. They beat us worse, 103–91.

Down 3–1 in the series and going back to L.A., it didn't look good for us. But that's where being a team of misfits worked in our favor. There was nothing typical about us, so we didn't expect things to go the way they did for anyone else. I'm sure the Lakers saw us complaining to the refs and arguing amongst ourselves and thought they had us down for the count. But we actually played better when we were doubted or had something to prove. It was when we were ahead or in control that we had a tendency to relax or get distracted. Win the next three games (two on the road and one at home) after losing two straight at home? No problem. We went back into Staples Center and did just that, winning 96–88. And now we had a chance to go back to the Rose Garden and set things right with our fans.

Shaq was still getting his fair share, but he was having to work for everything, and it started to show. Sabas, meanwhile, seemed to be finding a groove now that he wasn't in foul trouble. It all came together in Game 6. Shaq only had 17 points. Sabas was in his bag of tricks, scoring 10 points, grabbing 11 rebounds, and dishing out six assists. With Shaq not being his usual self, we outscored them by 20 in the paint and won the battle of the boards (43–34) for a 103–93 win.

I've never been so happy about going back to L.A. Now the Lakers were the ones staggering and we had every reason to believe we were about to hit them with a knockout blow.

It's still hard for me to talk about Game 7. The refs called two early fouls on Sabas, prompting Mike to sub me in for him with just under four minutes left in the first quarter to guard Shaq. Sixty seconds later, I was back on the bench after a pair of ticky-tack fouls. The defense they'd let me play all series long suddenly wasn't allowed. I didn't even get a chance to put a forearm in Shaq's ribs. I wanted to curse out the refs on my way back to the bench but I didn't want to look back and be the reason we'd lost by getting thrown out or for giving the refs a reason to dislike us more than they already did.

Jermaine came in for me and before the quarter was out they hit him with a foul, too. But Mike stayed with him and Jermaine came up with a couple of plays, blocking a shot by Kobe and drawing an offensive foul on Shaq.

Despite all the foul trouble, we were ahead for most of the first three quarters, going into the final period leading 71–58. The Staples Center might've been the Lakers' home floor, but we were playing as if we owned it.

I do remember sitting on the bench in the final seconds of the third quarter and thinking, *Oh, shit*. We were ahead by 16 when Brian Shaw threw up a three-point shot—and banked it in. You could feel a little spark of life blow back into them.

The spark, slowly but surely, became a fire, and damned if we could put it out. It started with Sabas picking up three fouls in about five minutes and fouling out. Mike might've brought me in to play Shaq in the final minutes, anyway, but now he had to bring me in way sooner than he would've wanted. He'd also left me on the bench since those first two early fouls and given my minutes to Detlef. I wasn't happy about not playing but we were winning and that's all that really mattered.

The fourth-quarter fouls allowed the Lakers to chip away at our lead from the free-throw line with the clock stopped. Meanwhile, we couldn't make a shot. Everybody kept shooting, trying to turn the momentum, instead of passing the ball and working our offense. The Lakers found their confidence and started talking shit and that's when all of us thought, *Oh, shit*.

The pace of an NBA game, especially in the playoffs, slows down in the fourth quarter and becomes a possession-by-possession battle. That gave the advantage to Shaq, because now I've had to keep him from backing me down under the rim every time down the floor. The difference in height and weight wore me down. It wouldn't have mattered if we could've kept scoring the way we did the first three quarters, but we were suddenly missing shots we'd made all year. I wasn't one of our big offensive weapons, but I wasn't going to let us go down without trying.

But I couldn't make anything, either. I drove to the hoop but Shaq swatted my shot. I took my next shot from one of my favorite spots, the left elbow of the free-throw line, but my shot banged off the backboard. Rasheed had been an offensive matchup nightmare for them and we got him the ball on his sweet spot, the left block, but the ball just wouldn't go down. Steve Smith, our best shooter, missed too. In the end, maybe that's what did us in—we had never established who our go-to guy was all season long. Sometimes it was Sheed, sometimes it was Steve, sometimes it was Scottie or Damon. So, with a championship on the line, we all tried on our own to be That Guy.

With Kobe and Shaq, the Lakers didn't have that problem. They knew where they wanted the ball to go—into Shaq—and if for some reason they couldn't get it there, then it was up to Kobe. Sometimes knowing exactly what you want to do under pressure is half the battle.

If you've ever watched highlights of the Kobe-Shaq era or an NBA commercial for the playoffs, you've seen the play that sealed our fate. If you look closely, you'll also see me in the middle of it.

The Lakers led 83–79 when Scottie missed a three-pointer with just under a minute left. Some teams might've focused on just taking time off the clock, but the Lakers were feeling good about themselves. Besides, Kobe had the ball and he was always going for the kill.

I remember the play like it was yesterday. Kobe turned the corner at the top of the key, got a step on Steve, and drove right down the lane. That left me with a choice—stay on Shaq, or step up and challenge Kobe, hoping somebody else would slide over and guard Shaq. Kobe with the ball and a clear look at the basket, it doesn't matter where he was, you had to be thinking he would shoot—either a floater or maybe go all the way to the rim and dunk it. So I ran out at him and hoped somebody down low would back me up. But nobody did.

Kobe saw me leave Shaq and made the right play, tossing the ball up near the rim. With no one to put a body on him, Shaq had a free run to the basket. All he had to do was jump, snag the ball with one of his big mitts, and flush it through the hoop.

Which he did.

Imagine if you had a nightmare and somehow someone was able to record it. And every time you turned on your TV, they were showing your nightmare. That's what that Kobe/Shaq lob dunk, followed by Shaq running down the court with a look of disbelief and Kobe yelling, "Our game!" is for me. Maybe if I'd stayed on Shaq and let Kobe score, he wouldn't have been so animated. But Shaq ran his ass down the court screaming, "Ahhhhhhh!"

To this day, I think, *Yeah, you dunked it. You should have with nobody on you!*

The NBA included that play in a commercial promoting the playoffs. I'm pretty sure they're still showing it. I have people tell me all the time, "Hey, I saw you on TV. Shaq was dunking on you." And I think to myself, *Yeah, great. Thanks.*

We were probably cooked the second Kobe found his way into the paint. But I knew one play could change everything and I was still hoping I could make it. That's the nightmare. Some people find themselves running in mud with a monster bearing down on them. Or tied down, unable to move, and some snaggle-toothed, foul-smelling beast breathing in their face. Mine is being stuck, helpless, between two Hall of Famers about to crush my dream of going to the NBA Finals.

No one said anything in the locker room. It was as if we'd all been knocked unconscious and woke up in the locker room and said, "What happened?" I looked around and thought, *This is over. This team is done.* I just knew this would be the last time I'd see this group together. This had been our shot and we all knew it. No one was sure what Whitsitt would do, but it was guaranteed he'd do something. And if anybody had a reason to wonder if he'd be back, it was me.

chapter 9

Taking My Talents to South Beach

Portland had become home. It *felt* like home. The people didn't put on airs and they respected hard work. If you were good to them, they were good to you. The outdoors and fishing were right up my alley. The long months of rain and cold were tougher on Gina because she had to take care of the house and the family while I was off playing in Florida and Texas and California getting a sunshine break, but we made a lot of good friends and the pace of life was good for both of us.

As I got on the team plane back home from L.A. after that heartbreaking loss to the Lakers, though, I knew I had to figure out where I wanted to play next. Because it wasn't going to be in Portland.

My agent had found out that Whitsitt intended to trade me for a power forward he'd had a lot of success with in Seattle and knew extremely well: the Reign Man, Shawn Kemp.

That might not have been all that bad if Shawn were still with the Sonics, but he wasn't. He'd spent the last three seasons with the Cleveland Cavaliers, traded there by the GM who replaced Whitsitt, Wally Walker. The Cavs also had a GM who knew me extremely well: Jim Paxson, who had been an assistant GM with the Blazers before going to Cleveland.

I had nothing against Jim or the Cavaliers, but I had no interest in going back to Ohio. Knowing Whitsitt, neither Mark nor I expected that to stop him from dealing me there.

As GM of the Sonics, Whitsitt had drafted Shawn and watched him develop into a six-time All-Star and help lead the Sonics to the place the Blazers had failed to reach with me—the Finals. Shawn had signed with the Cavaliers for the big contract he'd always wanted but struggled once he got there. The Cavs were looking to deal him for someone with the toughness and work ethic that fans in northeastern Ohio appreciated: me.

When Gina heard that we might be going to Cleveland, she cast her vote pretty quickly.

"Let's just stay in Portland," she said.

I had to explain to her that Whitsitt was known as "Trader Bob" for a reason, and that not opting out of my contract or signing a new one with the Blazers wouldn't guarantee I would stay with them; all it would do is give Whitsitt control over where he wanted to send me. That I was a native Buckeye only made it that much more appealing—to the Cavs. I loved Cleveland the city and community, but I knew that playing that close to home wasn't everything some make it out to be. It's not like high school or even college, where friends and family are just there to support you. When you turn pro and if you are easily accessible, that can be a challenge. Everyone and anyone I'd ever crossed paths with growing up would want tickets, a favor, a loan, or something, and I'm not good at saying no or disappointing people. I'd had a conversation with Damon Stoudamire when he first arrived in Portland; he'd been born and went to high school there.

"Man, how you like it?" I asked

"It's cool," he said. But a few years later, he had changed his mind. "Man, I might've made a mistake," he said.

The Cavs were also rebuilding, which meant more losing than I wanted to experience at that point in my career. The New York Knicks were interested as well and I would've gone there, even though I'm sure it would've been a rollercoaster. As much as I fed off people doubting me, Knicks' fans and the New York media are in a class of their own. I would've needed some thick skin. It didn't matter, though, because they didn't have anybody Whitsitt was willing to take in a trade. That meant Mark and I had to find a good team that needed a power forward and had the financial room to pay me at least something close to what I could make in Cleveland. A place with good weather would be nice, too.

That, obviously, was a tall order. It was also a nerve-wracking process, not knowing where we were going to live, who I was going to play for, and what I was going to get paid. That's a lot of unknowns and a lot of stress. Gina and I decided to go to Jamaica on vacation, hoping it would clear our heads and allow us to figure out what was most important to us.

When Mark heard where we were going, he asked if we'd stop in Miami on the way.

"Why?" I asked.

"I'd like you to meet with Pat Riley," Mark said.

That only sounded slightly better than going to Cleveland. The Heat were good and Riley was a coaching legend. He started his career leading Magic and Kareem and the Showtime Lakers to four championships (1982, '85, '87, '88) and four consecutive Finals' appearances (1982–85). Then he'd gone to New York and taken the Knicks to the Finals for the first time in 21 years, before going down to take over the Heat. He knew what it took to build a winning team and a winning culture.

He was also a legend for making players work harder than they ever had in their lives—and grinding a few years off their careers in the process. I was not afraid of working hard, but with all the injuries I'd had to deal with and play through, I wasn't sure my body would hold up to playing for the man.

"I don't know," I told Mark.

"We're not committing to anything," Mark said. "Just go see him."

Coach, as I like to call him, was our personal tour guide through the brand-new home the Heat were building, American Airlines Arena. At one point he raised the blinds on one side of the arena, providing a spectacular view of South Beach, the area famous for its night life.

"If you come here you won't be seeing much of that," he said. He was right. There were times the blinds were up and I'd ask to have them drawn. Seeing what was out there and knowing I was not going to have the energy to check it out became torture.

He also told me on that visit they only had a salary slot to pay me $2.25 million. It's not the sales pitch most coaches would make, but Riles was different. I had just spent a year coming off the bench and played less than eight minutes in Game 7 of the Western Conference finals, but he was pumping me up as if I'd just led the Blazers to a championship.

"We've only got $2.25 but this is where I see you playing," he said. "We're missing what you could give us. We need it. We think you would be just perfect. You've probably heard rumors. We don't work that hard, but we work. Millions of dollars are changing hands and I owe it to my owner to make sure we get the most out of our players."

I told him I'd actually heard his workouts were pretty rigorous.

"As hard as you work, they won't bother you," he said. "They only bother guys who don't like to work."

It wasn't the arena or the scenery or even the talent on the team that got me. What got me was him. His confidence. I ate it up.

I told him I'd take the $2.25 million and that I was coming to Miami.

After we got back from Jamaica, Gina and I went to visit everybody in Georgetown. The Cavs were not giving up. Paxson flew down to Cincinnati to meet with me and personally offer a max deal of $92 million over seven years.

When Riley heard about the offer, he called me while I was still in Ohio. "What are you going to do?" he asked.

"Well, I gave you my word I was coming to play for you," I said. "So I'm coming to Miami."

Even he thought I had to be out of my mind. "Are you for real?"

"I might be crazy, but yeah, that's what I'm doing."

"Alright, just hang in there," he said. "You sure you don't want to go on vacation again? They're going to be wearing you out." I think he was worried I might realize how much money I was sacrificing and change my mind.

"No, we're going to go back home," I said. I did tell him I could use a techno gym bike so I could work out at home, what with the Blazers' facilities not being available to me and figuring I might get some backlash working out in public somewhere. The bike arrived at my house in Portland before we did.

Word about my plan to go to Miami beat us back to Portland as well. We got off the plane and everyone started surrounding Gina and me as we walked through the terminal saying, "Hey, man, don't go." A little old lady came up and said, "You're such a good role model for my grandson. Will you please just stay here? We want you to stay." I looked at Gina and she had tears in her eyes, which made all of it hit twice as hard. We had to walk through a crowd of Blazers' fans, wait what seemed like forever at the baggage carousel for our luggage, and then walk past all those sad faces again. That was tough.

The local columnists and reporters weren't quite as nice. They either wrote that I was the dumbest person alive to pass on the kind of money the Cavs were offering or suspected I had some sort of back-room deal with the Heat that assured me of more money down the line. I'm confident the Heat would've taken care of me eventually, but there were no promises like that made; I'd tell you if they had. They were offering nothing more than $2.25 million for one year. I know how crazy it sounds to turn down $92 million for that, but it was perfectly clear to me—I couldn't stay in Portland, I didn't want to go to Cleveland, Whitsitt wouldn't trade me to New York, so Miami was my only option. I suppose a part of me figured I'd find a way to make that money at some point. But Gina knew there was no back-room deal and even she had her doubts about turning down Cleveland. "That's a lot of money," she said. "I hope you know what you're doing."

When Whitsitt heard I wouldn't accept the Cavs' offer, he figured he had me cornered and made another offer, promising he'd keep me in Portland.

"No, I made a commitment to Pat and I'm going to keep it," I said.

"You're going to turn this down for that?" Whitsitt said. "Well, you know, good luck to you." And he hung up.

The day before I could officially sign, Riley called. "You still coming?" he asked.

"Yeah," I said.

"It's been tough, huh?"

"Yeah. A lot of people are calling me ignorant and stupid, but I'm a man of my word. I've been working out on the techno bike. I've lost weight."

"Alright. You're a man of your word."

Mark called me the next day. "You're not going to believe the deal that Riley made so you can get paid," he said. The Cavs were even a key part of it. Whitsitt was still determined to get Kemp, so he agreed to be part of a three-team trade between the Cavaliers, Blazers, and Heat. The league's salary cap rules were devised by a roomful of lawyers and that becomes pretty clear to anyone who has read them. Or tried to follow them. Teams at that time were allowed to go over the salary cap to re-sign their own players, even if they planned to immediately trade them. It's known in the business as a "sign-and-trade" and that's what the Blazers did with me. Riley gave up a future first-round pick and two players—Clarence Weatherspoon and Chris Gatling—just so I could play for him on a seven-year, $86 million deal rather than $2.25 million. And Whitsitt got Shawn.

"You were a man of your word," Riley said, "and I rewarded you for that."

What stays with me is that he didn't have to do it. He already had a loaded team and I didn't have any other options. At least none that I was willing to take. I would've played, hoped to have a good year, and then hit the market again. I'm glad I didn't have to go that route because even with the bigger paycheck, Riles made sure to get his money's worth out of me.

He warned me about the conditioning test that everybody had to pass the first day of training camp. It's called "Tens." As in 10 lengths of the court. Guards had to do it in 60 seconds, wings in 63 seconds, and big men in 65 seconds.

Oh, and you had to do five of them in all. The only good part is that you could bank your extra seconds. So let's say I ran my first "Ten" in 59 seconds, now I had six seconds in the bank. If I did the second one in 60 seconds, now I've banked another five seconds, so I've got 11 seconds in the bank. If my legs started to get heavy and burn with the third one and it took me 63 seconds, that's still another two seconds in the bank for 13. The fourth one, if I finished in 66 seconds, now I just had to do the last one in 77 seconds (65+12). At that point, something crazy would have to happen for me not to make it.

If you didn't pass, though, you had to do it the next day, and every day after that until you made it. I went down to Miami early to get ready and I'm glad I did. Bill Foran, the strength & conditioning coach, prepared those of us who were in town by timing us while we did "Tens" several times a week. He built us up from one to a set of three and that was hard enough. I wasn't sure how I'd do five, but I did. Everybody was coughing up a lung by the end; then we stretched and went right into practice, which included a drill where we ran down the sidelines, pivoted, and then ran backward with our hands up the entire time. The most the players union allowed teams to practice at that time was four hours a day and Pat had us coming in every day right under four hours. He had his blue cards, the entire practice written out, minute by minute. Players around the league heard all about it. Everybody I knew at some point said, "Man, I feel bad for you." We'd go home so tired, no one had any interest in going to South Beach. We'd play with the kids a bit and then lay down.

I didn't have a problem with it. I grew up with an appetite for anything physical; I actually enjoyed it. I was a pre-teen when I started working with my grandfather, cutting tobacco, baling hay, digging potatoes, and picking beans. That's hard-ass work, all of it. I believe that's where I developed my resilience, because if you can cut a quarter mile of tobacco, you can do basically anything.

I also like to eat, which was a big bonus for working on someone's farm. We were only paid a couple of bucks an hour. There was an old guy, 75 or so, who would hire us when it was harvest time. He'd ride around on his tractor and tell us what he wanted done. When it was time for lunch he'd bring us all up to his country house. His wife would lay out a spread of pork chops, fried chicken, mashed potatoes, green beans, kale, and cherry pie. We'd eat and then be ready for a nap, but we still had another half-day's work in the field. Guys playing basketball talk about "being on their grind" when they go through multiple workouts in a day; trust me, there's no grind like working all day in the fields.

What I didn't like were the snakes, although they probably helped develop my hops, because if I saw one in the tobacco fields you could bet I was leaving my feet.

For training camp, we stayed in a hotel north of the city. It was just the players, but family could come visit. We had a curfew and everything. It was Riley's show. I was coming from Portland, which was basically the Wild West, so it took a little adjusting. But there was purpose and rationale behind everything Riley did. You could drop him in the middle of a hurricane and everybody would be laid out and he'd come out standing, because that's how he is.

Living off the court in Miami was a lot different than Portland, too. I talked to my neighbors all the time in Portland; in Miami, depending on where you lived, you might not even know who your neighbors were. Gina became friends with the wives of players who had houses in Miami but didn't play for the Heat. It was a culture shock, too. I wasn't used to being around so many people speaking Spanish, and not slow Spanish, either. But for the most part everything took a backseat to playing for the Heat. There was never a day off—you were doing something every day, even if the team didn't practice together. I respected Riley for that. You were going to learn to be a professional playing for him or you were going to run a hell of a lot of sprints. Or you were going to be gone.

Luckily, I was going to have help meeting Riley's expectations. I didn't know it at the time, but my battles with Karl Malone had caught the attention of a Miami-based personal trainer, Dodd Romero.

Glen Rice, who started his career with the Heat and still lived in Miami during the off-season, threw a little party at his house not long after I arrived. When Gina and I got there, Glen said, "My boy, Dodd, wants to meet you."

Glen pointed him out to me and I walked over, stuck out my hand, and said, "I'm Brian."

"Dodd, pleased to meet you, pleased," he said and then walked by me.

I went back to Glen and told him what happened. "What's wrong with him?" I asked.

"Oh, that's just Dodd. He wanted me to tell you to meet him at his gym tomorrow at one o'clock."

"Man, I'm not working out with that guy. He's going to get me all big."

"You don't have to work out with him," Glen said. "Just meet him."

Dodd wouldn't talk to me, but he brought his wife, Sabina, over to explain why he wanted to meet me.

"Dodd can't tell the story because he gets too pumped up and then he has to go work out for two hours," she said. "All because of you."

"What'd I do?"

Dodd started to butt in and then butted out. "Tell him," he said to Sabina. "I'm going to go over here." A few minutes later he's yelling across the room, "Okay, what part are you at?"

Sabina told me she had been clicking through TV channels in search of something to watch and then handed the remote to Dodd and left the room. A minute later, Dodd called her back.

"Hey, baby. Come here. Look at this guy out here battling Karl Malone." It was the game where Dunleavy got thrown out and I acted as if I was going to throw the ball at Karl for a split-second and then we wound up in each other's face with me talking junk and Karl just taking it all in.

"Sabina, God just told me I'm going to train him some day," Dodd said.

"What? You don't even know him."

Dodd jumped up. "I can't watch it no more," he said and, as Sabina tells it, he went to the gym and put in a two-hour workout to burn off the adrenaline boost he got from watching me and Karl go at it.

We did meet the day after Glen's party, but we didn't work out much; instead, we traded stories about how we'd ended up where we were and felt as if some divine power had been at work. I told him about Mr. Martt, the persistent anonymous caller to Xavier, slipping in under the change in admissions requirements, and getting placed with two great lob-throwing guards at the Desert Classic.

His stories were even more extraordinary, but anyone who knows Dodd would not find that surprising. This is a guy who likes to challenge himself by wrestling wild animals. His list includes a rhino, a zebra, a bear, and an alligator. The alligator was in the wild and he had to swim up under it, in murky swamp water no less. He has no interest in hurting them; he says he only wants to put them in submission and let them feel his and God's love and then let them go.

Sabina was not aware that when they went to a zoo on their first date he had been banned from about 20 of them for climbing into various animal's pens to wrestle them. When he showed her how to sneak into the zoo by hopping a fence, she knew he was crazy. When she followed him over the fence, Dodd told me later, he knew he'd found his wife.

Once inside, they passed a sign that said, "New Exhibit: The Komodo Dragon." Dodd abruptly asked Sabina if she'd go buy them a couple of Pepsis. She suspected something was up because even though they hadn't known each other all that long, she was already aware Dodd followed a pretty strict diet and didn't drink anything with sugar in it. But after some coaxing, she went. As soon as she was out of sight, apparently, he went over the rail.

Sabina was on her way back with the sodas when she heard loud hissing sounds from the exhibit. Dodd had repelled down the side of the wall into a moat, swam across it, and was slowly approaching the dragon. Now, he knew his animals; he was well aware that one bite from a Komodo dragon could kill him. I would tell you the technique for grabbing a dragon without getting bitten, but I don't know it. Dodd, however, apparently did, because, with Sabina watching, he was able to get on top and hold it so the dragon couldn't twist its head to bite him. She could hear him talking to the dragon as he positioned his hands to stroke its head, saying softly, "Settle down. Settle down." When he let go, the dragon ran over to the far side of the enclosure and Dodd got back across the moat and climbed back up the wall.

"I knew you were going to wrestle that thing," Sabina told him.

"Well, I'm glad you didn't interrupt me," he said. "I could've died."

What made Dodd a true believer is a series of events that saved his daughter's life. His daughter, Gianna, was born with a vein on the wrong side of her liver. It kept her sick through much of her childhood. When she was hospitalized and the doctors told Dodd she was going to die without a liver transplant, Dodd spent the next three days in church, praying, "Lord, give me my baby girl back and I will never put another drink in my body again and I will serve you the rest of my life."

Dodd had started working as a personal trainer in high school. He did it for free for classmates who wanted to be wrestlers or football players.

One day, a classmate came up to him and said, "I want to play football. How much can I pay you to get me right?"

Dodd could've taken the guy's money, but he knew the guy just didn't have the physique to play football. "You're not ever going to play football," he said. "You don't have the body for it. Go be a doctor or a lawyer."

Fast forward to Dodd now being a full-time personal trainer. He was in the gym and noticed a guy having a problem with one of his hands. The man saw Dodd looking at him and said, "I'm a surgeon. I had to quit my practice because of this."

"I can fix that," Dodd said.

"Yeah, right," the former surgeon said. "I have a medical degree. I can't tell you how many specialists I've seen. This can't be fixed."

"I don't operate on their level," Dodd said. "I operate on the Lord's level. If you want your hand to be fixed, it can be fixed."

The surgeon had nothing to lose. He started to train with Dodd and sure enough, Dodd restored the dexterity and flexibility in his hand and the surgeon was able to get his license back.

After the three days of prayer, Dodd gets notified that they've found a liver for Gianna. Who is the medic that delivers the new liver? The wanna-be football player Dodd told to study medicine. Who is the surgeon that replaces Gianna's old liver with the new one? The one whose hand function Dodd restored.

This is the man who said to me that first day we met in his gym, "We're going to be brothers for life, like blood brothers. Even closer."

Dodd's spiritual support was almost as important as his training tips, because not long after I got to Miami, my friend Miguel Reyes' daughter, Jovita, had to undergo hip surgery. All of the cancer treatment had left her bones far more fragile than they normally would be for a young girl. In the operating room, they realized that her entire system had been compromised. She bled out in surgery. The following summer, Dodd went with me back to Oregon to have a celebration of life to remember Jovita and, upon meeting Miguel and learning of his Native American heritage, announced that we were staying to build a sweat lodge so we could all sweat together. Which we did.

That season would've been a tough one even without losing Jovita. As I got ready for training camp, I looked at our roster and thought, "We are about to roll over people." We had All-Star talent at every position: Alonzo Mourning at center, Eddie Jones at shooting guard, and Tim Hardaway at point guard. Neither I nor Anthony "Mase" Mason had been All-Stars but we had back-ups who had been, Cedric Ceballos and A.C. Green.

Then training camp started and one day Coach announced that Zo was retiring because he'd been diagnosed with a rare kidney disease. The next thing he said was, "Brian, you need to play center." I had lost more than 10 pounds getting in shape to handle Riley's conditioning demands, so now I was going to be at even more of a physical disadvantage playing Shaq, Sabas, and just about every other center. This wasn't going to be relief duty, either, the way it had been with the Blazers. I was going to get their best shot for 35 minutes a night. (Now you know why I was willing to let Philippe stick his needles in me.) But I hadn't forgot what Riley had done to get me my contract. I was still ready to go to war for him.

The schedule gave me an early chance to prove it. The fifth game of the season we went back to one of my favorite places on earth, Salt Lake City, and beat the Jazz. I led us in scoring with 21 and rebounds with 10.

A week later, the Blazers came to town. Detlef and Jermaine had left, but they'd added Kemp and center Dale Davis, who was coming off his lone All-Star season with the Indiana Pacers. They were still loaded.

We were anything but loaded at the moment. Besides Zo, we were missing our starting backcourt, Eddie and Tim. Dan Majerle, Eddie's back-up, was out, too. I don't know what the odds were, but we went into the game as major underdogs. In other words, I was in my sweet spot. Pat put the lineups on the white board in the locker room and it was one mismatch after another in favor of the Blazers. Was I confident we were going to win? Hell, yeah, I was.

Everybody was out there hugging before the tipoff, but once we got started I went after Sheed hard. "Damn, BG!" he said.

"No, no, no, we're not friends right now," I said. One time, Shawn, Sabonis, and I all went up for the rebound of a missed shot at our basket. I got it and stuck it back in and as I ran back on defense I let their bench know all about it.

Shawn and Sabas probably weren't too happy, but the Blazers' bench mob loved it. "Go take your crazy ass down the court!" one of them shouted. It didn't stop there. Every time I got the ball down low I was going up with it. We ended up winning, 86–80. I led all scorers and rebounders with 24 points and 13 rebounds. Had a couple of blocked shots, too. We met on the court afterward and several of them said, "Man, we miss you." That meant a lot. "I miss you all, too, but I'm digging it down here," I said. "It's cool."

It was just a regular-season game, but it has a spot in my heart right next to my battles with the Lakers and with Karl. I get pumped all over again just thinking about it.

Individual honors were never something that motivated me, but I thought I might have a shot at being an All-Star that season. Zo was voted in as a starter by the fans even though he wasn't playing. The coaches picked the reserves, and that's where I thought I had a chance. Theo Ratliff from the Philadelphia 76ers and Dikembe Mutombo with the Atlanta Hawks were the other Eastern Conference centers chosen. Theo missed the game with an injury, so the league had to pick replacements for him and Zo. I started the season off well, but by January I was struggling and Mase picked up the slack. He and Antonio Davis from the Toronto Raptors were selected as the Eastern

Conference replacements. It didn't bother me much then. I wanted to get the job done in front of me, whatever my coach decided that was. Now? Sure, I wish I had at least one All-Star appearance on my résumé, but at the time I was happy to get the weekend off to rest.

Zo found treatment for his kidney that allowed him to come back and play the final 13 games of the season and we cruised into the playoffs as the No. 3 seed in the Eastern Conference. That, however, lined us up with the sixth-seeded Charlotte Hornets. They were a mini-version of my old Blazers' team, with swagger for days, thanks to point guard Baron "B-Diddy" Davis and Jamal Mashburn. "Styles make fights," they say, and their run-and-gun style was way too much for us. Besides, Mash had been with the Heat and was traded to the Hornets before the season for Eddie and Mase, so he had some revenge in mind.

With Zo back and Mase an All-Star, I came off the bench. They swept us out of the playoffs in three games that weren't close. Mash was far and away the best player in the series, averaging almost 24 points, six rebounds, and nearly five assists for the three games.

My second season I finally got a chance to do what I expected when I arrived in Miami—start at power forward next to Zo. But he wasn't the only one that had me excited about being part of the Heat when I arrived. I came there looking forward to playing with Zo *and* Hardaway, Eddie, and Majerle. That never happened. We were way too expensive for a first-round-and-out team. The team had to get rid of a few salaries, which meant getting rid of some talent. Hardaway was traded to the Dallas Mavericks for a future second-round pick. Mase and Majerle were both free agents; Mase signed a four-year deal with the Milwaukee Bucks and Majerle went back to his first team, the Phoenix Suns, for a one-year retirement tour.

There was one other problem: Zo and I were at our best playing around the basket, but with both of us starting, there was only room for one. There was never a doubt who that would be—Zo. But he wasn't the same Zo I had battled as a King or Blazer. He could still block shots and he played as hard as ever, but he had slowed down a lot. I wasn't quite the same, either. Looking back, I realize now that first year at center took something out of me I never got back. I had slimmed down and prepared myself to outrun every power forward in the league. The move to center meant being in the trenches, trying to hold off guys 50 or 60 pounds heavier on a nightly basis. It was like training to run the 40 in a track meet and then being told you've been switched to sumo wrestling.

With Zo in the low post, I had to play at the high post or the short corner on offense, taking more jumpers but fewer shots overall. It also meant not as many chances to get points and rebounds off put-backs of missed shots. Or draw fouls, since the cardinal rule in basketball is not to foul a jump shooter.

We knew we might struggle out of the gate, but it was worse than that: we lost 23 of our first 28 games. Our season was unofficially over by New Year's Eve. Except that with Riley, there was never a reason to throw in the towel. Our conditioning and attention to detail eventually began to pay off and we climbed to within four games of a winning record. If we could climb over .500, we still had a shot at making the playoffs.

Pat had never coached a team to a losing record or one that didn't make the playoffs in 19 seasons with three different franchises—the Lakers, the Knicks, and the Heat. We were the lowest scoring team in the league, but Coach figured we could overcome that by being the best defensive team. All that took was effort, discipline, and conditioning.

It wasn't enough. We didn't break 90 in 12 of our last 20 games; we scored less than 80 in five of them. For the last month, we never won two games in a row.

As frustrating as that season might have been for all of us, the next season proved to be even worse. Zo's kidney problems surfaced again and he missed the entire season. Caron Butler, a rookie small forward, played more minutes than anybody. We had another slow start, losing 15 of our first 20 games, but this time it never got better. From January 1 until the end of the season, we never had a winning streak. We'd win a game, then lose three, win another one and lose four more.

It killed me that we weren't doing better or that I couldn't do more. I tried to make up for it by making myself available, no matter how I felt physically, and played all 82 games for the first and only time in my career, even though I had bone on bone in my right knee. The way we were playing wasn't translating into wins and me being out there every night wasn't making much of a difference, but I would've felt a lot worse sitting on the bench watching us lose. Besides, we had a mix of older guys all struggling to stay healthy and a bunch of young guys who were just figuring out the NBA game. I'd go around to everybody's locker after practices and games, trying to keep both the rookies and old vets believing we could turn it around, and the only way my word would mean anything is if I was right there going through the hard times with them.

I needed a lot of help to do that. I had Philippe with his massages and acupuncture needles at home after games and the entire Heat medical staff working on me just about every day before and after practice. I spent so much time in the training room, the staff felt like family. I looked at Ron Culp (the head athletic trainer) and Dr. Harlan Selesnik (the team doctor and orthopedic surgeon) as my uncles, and assistant athletic trainer Jay Sabol and masseuse Vinny Aquillino as my brothers.

What I remember as much as anything from that season was being on a training table every morning to have them work on my knee, with Eddie on the table next to me, getting work on his ankle or groin.

I'm confident in saying we were the hardest working 25-win team ever. If the end of the previous season was a punch to the gut for Coach, this one took him over the edge. The league fined him a bunch of times for complaining about the officiating in his postgame press conferences.

With about 10 games left, we were officially eliminated from playoff contention. Coach walked into the gym that day and said, "We mathematically can't make it to the playoffs. But we owe it to the owners, the fans, and the organization to still work, work, work, work, work hard."

So even though we were eliminated, Pat still had us practicing the full four hours allowed. "Killer 17s" might be as bad as "Tens," if not worse. You have to run 17 times from sideline to sideline in under a certain time. Pat's was 70 seconds for everybody. Any time anybody made a mistake, Pat would bark, "On the line. 17." We ran at least five or six every practice, along with a lot of other conditioning drills. It got to the point where our wives were talking to each other about how beat up we were coming home. I overheard Gina one day talking to Eddie Jones' wife.

"Eddie can't move," Trina Jones said.

"Brian comes home and just lays on the couch," Gina said. "Some nights he sleeps there because he can't get up the stairs."

Most of us saw it as a challenge, a test to see who was in and who was out, when it came to believing in Coach. By now we had all lost another five or six pounds of lean muscle. I knew Eddie and me were in, but his ankle was swelling up really bad and I was having the same problem with my knee.

Finally, Culp walked up to Pat and said, "You can't keeping doing this. You're not going to give up and neither are Eddie or Brian and they're going to hurt themselves. It's not worth it."

We lined up, waiting for him to tell us to go. He kept walking back and forth, looking at his notes. He looked up at me and then back at his notes. Then he looked at Eddie and back at his notes. Finally, he said, "Everybody go home," and he walked out.

We looked at each other. For a good part of the year, in Coach's pre-practice talks with us, I could tell he was searching for what to say or how to motivate us. It was as if he was wondering if his approach could still work or if he needed to change it up. But nothing like this had ever happened before. Assistant coach Stan Van Gundy and the rest of the staff rushed us out of the gym, worried, maybe, that Pat might change his mind. "Go, go, get out of here," they said. I don't even think any of us showered; we all hobbled into the locker room, changed out of our practice gear, and went home.

When we came in the next day, I figured with the day off he'd really run us hard. We all gathered on the practice court and after a minute or two, he said, "Go home" again. He walked off without saying another word.

We knew by then Coach was at a place he'd never been before—a place of uncertainty about what to do. You could tell he was looking at himself, questioning whether his methods still worked. I hated to see it. This was my coach, a man I admired, loved, and had the utmost respect for and was ready to follow, no questions asked. The third day was exactly the same, in that Coach came in and then told us we could go; only this time after he left, Van Gundy gathered us all together. "Listen, you know Pat's going through something," he said. "We're all going through something, but we take care of each other. So let's do our walk-through so we're prepared for the game."

When he walked into training camp the following year and told us he was stepping away from coaching and Stan would be taking over, I bawled my eyes out. That's how you know you love someone. As many times as I leaned against the wall, trying to catch my breath before having to run another "Tens" or "Killer 17s" and cussing him out under my breath, I always had a deep appreciation for the man. Even though he pushed me, he pushed me for a reason. He wanted me to believe in myself as much as he believed in me. I know other players had a different experience with him. People would ask me, "What horror story do you have?"

My answer: "Unless working hard for your money is a horror story, I don't have one." I meant it. My college workouts were the hardest I ever had until I got to Miami. No coach ever made me work harder than Pat. But no one was ever as loyal, either. If you're loyal to him, he'll go to bat for you in anything, in any way he can. Long after I stopped playing, he continued to prove that.

He wasn't always a straight taskmaster, either. There was only one kind of gym shoe I ever remember Pat wearing—the Nike Cortez. He loved that shoe and every few weeks it seemed as if he had on a fresh pair straight out of the box. If you remember that shoe, the sole had these deep ridges and the new ones could stick a little bit. Eddie House, one of our shooting guards, was always on the lookout for when Pat had new ones, because there would be a point where one of the soles would catch and he'd trip. "Pat forgot those things had grip," Eddie would whisper. That would get us both to laughing, but we'd have to hide it from Pat. After a while, though, Pat must've caught on because we'd catch him trying to hide that he was laughing, too.

As a player, I had learned how to regroup after a bad season or setback. There was never a thought of not playing anymore. I had to believe Pat was the same way with coaching. He didn't believe in giving in or giving up. So after all these years, for him to get to a point where he felt he had to stop, I could only imagine how hard that must've been. The only reason he would do it is because he felt he wasn't delivering on his promise to the players in exchange for what he was asking them to give. That had to be tough to accept for someone who had been as consistently successful as Pat.

The season under Stan didn't start out much different than the previous two. For three seasons in a row, we had the hardest time winning games in November. But this time it felt different. We started off 0–7 before getting our first win against the Cleveland Cavaliers and their No. 1 pick, LeBron James. Despite all the losing, Stan kept showing us statistically how we were playing better than our record might suggest.

It helped that we'd drafted a guard out of Marquette, Dwyane Wade. The first time we played some summer pick-up games at the arena, I clapped for the ball three or four times and he ignored me every time. "Hey, man," I said, "pass the goddamn ball sometimes."

Wade didn't blink. "Coach told me if I'm open, shoot," he said. "So I'm going to shoot."

I shook my head. I might've cursed him a little under my breath, but that still didn't stop him from shooting the ball every time he touched it. Between him, Eddie, and a young free agent small forward we signed, Lamar Odom, I accepted that shots were going to be hard to find. But then I was also back to playing center full-time again. Zo had recovered once more from his kidney issues but had decided to sign with the New Jersey Nets.

I also had a young rookie named Udonis Haslem pushing me. At this point I was just trying to get through practice, but U.D., as an undrafted free agent, was trying to prove he belonged and went at me every chance he had. I admired his hustle, but I warned him that one day he'd be in my shoes and some young buck would come along and make his life miserable just like he was trying to do to me. Sure enough, a few years ago I ran in to him and he said, "B, you were right. These boys are trying to dunk on me just like I tried to dunk on you."

Zo leaving left us with the money to sign Lamar, who was looking for a fresh start after starting his career with the Los Angeles Clippers. Riley believed in discipline and total dedication, but he also made up his own mind about people. He would take a chance on a guy if he saw something good in them and thought they could give the team something it didn't have.

Lamar, as anyone will tell you, is a good dude; he just got caught up in doing some things that knocked him off track. I didn't understand the demons he was dealing with then as I do now, but I never doubted his heart or his talent. He was apparently nervous about fitting in with us, so Pat asked us to welcome him. A few of us scooped him up after his introductory press conference. Riley asked us to give Lamar a fresh start and accept him as one of us. It didn't take much convincing because we knew how good he was.

Overall, it was a good fit between Stan and the players—we all had something to prove, one way or the other, and we were all willing to help each other. Stan was getting a chance to be a head coach for the first time. Dwyane wanted to prove he could be a star. I still wanted to prove Pat right for bringing me to Miami, in spite of how the previous two seasons had gone. We had several veteran players who felt that way. And Lamar wanted to prove he could be part of a winning organization.

By December, all that synergy started to pay off. We had a winning month, 8–7! March is when we really took off, winning 12 of 15 games. We finished with a winning record, 42–40, and earned the fourth seed in the Eastern Conference playoffs, with our first-round opponent being the fifth-seeded Hornets. They had moved to New Orleans, but they still had most of the guys who had crushed us three years earlier, including Jamal Mashburn and Baron Davis. We went a full seven games, with the home team winning every game—which meant we got our revenge and moved on to face the Indiana Pacers.

The Pacers still had Reggie Miller, Metta World Peace (when he was still Ron Artest), and my former Blazer teammate, Jermaine O'Neal, who had become a full-fledged All-Star. We took two games off of them before our youth and overall lack of experience finally cost us, but we all went into the summer feeling as if we were back on the right track. I know I certainly did. I was looking forward to my fifth year in a Heat uniform being my most successful. Before we got halfway through the summer, though, I realized I'd better start looking forward to something somewhere else.

chapter 10
Breaking Down

Every summer my family would get together back in Georgetown and have our version of the Fourth of July—a big barbecue with fireworks. We often waited until after the Fourth of July because they'd sell the fireworks half off and I'd load up on them. My dad had a friend who knew how to set off the ones you loaded into metal pipes and shot into the air.

Gina and I went to Georgetown a couple of weeks after the Pistons upset the Lakers to win the championship. I was talking with my dad and brother about how good I thought we—the Heat—were going to be the next season, when the news broke that the Lakers All-Star center, Shaquille O'Neal, wanted out of L.A. I didn't really care. If anything, I liked the idea of Kobe and Shaq splitting up, but after all I'd experienced with Jerry West and the 2000 Western Conference finals, the less I thought about them, the better. I was far more focused on where the Heat were headed.

"We've got a good team," I said. "If we get one more piece, we might just take the East."

Then the news came out where Shaq wanted to go—and Miami was on the list. Now I not only knew who the one piece could be for the Heat, I knew who they'd use to get that piece.

"Gina, time to pack our bags," I said. "We're getting traded."

"Did somebody say that?" she asked.

"No, but if Miami is one of the places Shaq wants to play next season, Pat is going to get him and they're going to need my salary to make the numbers match up." League rules require that the value of the player contracts involved in a trade have to be close to matching. Eddie, me, and Lamar were the only ones with big enough salaries to offset the $24 million Shaq was making a year. Trading Eddie didn't really make sense because he was a guard and could play next to Shaq more effectively than I could, so I figured Pat had little choice but to make me part of the deal.

Sure enough, on July 14, Riley traded me, Caron, Lamar, a future first-round pick, and a future second-round pick to the Lakers for Shaq. In one way, it was a relief, because I wasn't sure where I might end up. In the same way Coach had made a three-team deal to get me to Miami, I thought he might need to bring in a third team to make a deal work and I could wind up some place I did not want to be.

Not that playing for the Lakers was ever a dream of mine. Not with my history against them. Far from it. It had been four years since we'd lost that Game 7 but I still harbored a lot of feelings about it. The other nagging thought I had was they weren't getting the version of me that had battled them those seven games. I still had the will but not the way. I'd run the floor as hard as I could but now I wasn't going by anybody. My side-to-side quickness wasn't there, either, the way it once had been. Looking back, I also wonder if I was feeling the first effects of Parkinson's, because I could not explode off my left leg the way I once could. It wasn't just a loss of strength but a sense of feeling unsteady, as if I couldn't trust it. At the time I just chalked it up to getting old. But for the first time I was thinking my remaining playing days were numbered.

I didn't hold anything against Miami or Pat for trading me. I would've made the same move if I was in his position. That 25-win year we were playing in front of crowds that felt like 3,000 people in the building and after they traded for Shaq I think season tickets sold out in about two days.

Pat also wrote me a long letter afterward. He must've been on the road because it was on the back of a big envelope. He wrote how much he hated trading me and thanked me for my professionalism and sacrifice and said if I ever had an opportunity to come back to Miami, I would have a spot on the roster. He also included a card that said "Forever" on it. He wrote, "If you ever need me, just pull your 'forever' card and I'll be there." That's exactly what I did after I got diagnosed with Parkinson's.

My time in a Lakers' uniform didn't go much better than all my other experiences involving them. At 32, I was suddenly the old head on the team; Vlade Divac was also on the roster and he was 36, but he barely played. I played, but a lot less than I ever had before. I wasn't just a role player, I was a bit player.

The Staples Center was a strange place to play. The real Lakers fans are up in the top section of the arena. Those are the ride-or-die fans. Some fans in the lower bowl are with you no matter what, but there's some that are only with you when you're going good; when you're not, they're finding something else to do.

Don't get me wrong—I'm a big movie buff, so seeing the actors and actresses I'd watched since I was a kid in person watching me work was a trip. There were special moments, like when Jessica Alba sat next to the bench. But I don't know if they were *actually* watching me work, because the attention could flip to something off the court in a minute. We'd be in the middle of a game and a cheer would go up and it would be because the arena cameras showed someone famous walking to their seat or someone doing something goofy for attention in the stands. The game itself sometimes felt like a side show.

Even so, I had these anxiety attacks just driving to the arena thinking about playing in front of a whole list of Who's Who in the entertainment industry. That probably had as much to do with the fact that I couldn't do what I once could as a player. I never connected with Lakers' fans the way I did in Sacramento or Portland or Miami, and part of that certainly had to be because I just couldn't battle the way I once did. A neck injury in training camp ended any chance of me starting and chronic tendonitis in both knees limited my minutes overall.

Bottom line is, I never had the chance to win the Lakers' fans over as I had everywhere else.

You know who else seemed to be having anxiety attacks? Rudy Tomjanovich, our head coach. He coached some great players and won two championships when he was with the Houston Rockets, so I went into L.A. thinking I could learn a few things from him. I have nothing but respect for the man, but it wasn't the experience I thought it would be. One day, I went up for a rebound with Kobe Bryant. I got it and put it back for a score and I guess Kobe didn't like that, because he started going at me. It got pretty chippy between us until finally we squared off. Rudy jumped in between us and said, "Alright, that's enough." For those who don't know, Rudy was a star forward for the Rockets when he got sucker-punched in a game against the Lakers by their power forward, Kermit Washington. He never saw the punch coming and it not only ended his season, it nearly killed him.

"That will be enough of the two of you," Rudy said. "I was involved in an accident where I almost lost my life because somebody punched me, and I'll be damned if I'm going to have that happen here."

The only problem I had with all that is Rudy was only looking at me while he said all that. Which I pointed out to him. "You might want to look at both of us because fuck you," I said.

"Whoa," Rudy said.

I'm sure some of my resentment came from feeling as if I had to fight every day to be respected, but that didn't change the fact that I was lit. "Don't just be looking at me, dude. I'm not a punk. I'm not a young rookie up in here, man. I'll cuss your ass out."

Rudy tried to smooth it over. "No, I'm just saying I want you guys to calm down."

We got back to scrimmaging and I went up and got another rebound and Kobe was right there when I came down with it. He looked at me and then started laughing and that got me to laughing, too, and it was over.

That was Rudy's first season as Lakers coach and he didn't make it all the way through. That's what I mean about him sharing my anxiety. Even though we were winning (24–19), Rudy resigned, saying he was mentally and physically exhausted. I can't say anything negative about him other than the way he handled that situation with Kobe and me. When you have a problem with me and someone else, make sure you look at the other person at least once, not just me.

Playing with Kobe, overall, was the best experience I took away from that season. I learned right away why he was so good—because he put in the work. I had always prided myself on being the first one in the gym and the last one out on the teams I played for, but he had me beat on the Lakers and he lived almost an hour south in Orange County at the time. Of course, he would hop in the commuter lane and if the cops pulled him over they'd recognize him and let him go. More than once I thought, *Damn, I wish I could do that.*

Even though I wasn't getting the same playing time and could feel my body breaking down, I took pride in working out, especially when it came to spending time in the weight room. One day I was in there with Kobe and did a set on the lat pull-down machine. I had all but the last five plates loaded onto the machine and lifted the stack twice. I was kind of feeling myself and Kobe noticed. "Hey, you did that two times?" he asked.

"Yeah," I said.

"You mind if I do a set?"

"Be my guest."

He loaded up every plate on the machine and lifted all of them. Five times.

I nodded. Point made, I thought to myself.

I always thought he was a cool dude, but I had so much more respect for him after I saw how he trained. You weren't going to outwork him, and I'm used to outworking people. He wasn't having it, and that's probably why we got into it in practice that day. But I also think that's why we hit it off a little bit.

Rudy's assistant, Frank Hamblen, took over for him and we collapsed, going 10–29, finishing 11th in the Western Conference, a long way from a playoff spot. Meanwhile, the Heat had the best record in the Eastern Conference and went to the conference finals, losing in seven games to the Detroit Pistons. I had been telling those close to me: "If I could get back to Miami, I would," but I had two more years left on my contract. I couldn't see a way the Heat could take on my contract and I couldn't be sure I'd still be playing in two years.

What I didn't see coming was a by-product of the league's new collective bargaining agreement. The old one ended with the 2004–05 season, but this time the owners and players union had already made a lot of progress negotiating a new one before the old one expired. On July 30, a new six-year CBA was in place—and it included something called an "amnesty clause," which allowed teams to waive one player. They still had to pay the player whatever his contract was worth, but his salary no longer counted against the salary cap, the money a team was allowed to spend in any one year on player salaries.

Ten days after the new CBA was in place, the Lakers decided that they could make better use of $14 million a year than spending it on a power forward averaging 3.8 points and 3.7 rebounds a game. As in, me. So they thanked me for my contribution and cut me loose. I was now free to sign with any team I wanted for whatever they could afford while I still got paid by the Lakers. This felt the same as Xavier plucking me out of Georgetown High or the Kings taking a no-name power forward out of Xavier. The basketball universe was throwing me a bone. Pat had told me in his letter I had a spot with the team if I wanted it. I was determined to take him up on that. There was only one wrinkle: it had to happen fast.

The NBA calendar normally runs from July 1 to June 30, which means player contracts normally end on June 30. An agent who has a player with an expiring contract starts talking to teams well before that to figure out what and where his next contract might be. Mark did that for me with both the Blazers and Heat. My free agency this time, though, was a total surprise. The CBA negotiations pushed back the start of free agency to August 2, but since the Lakers didn't waive me until August 10, I hit the market after most teams had already filled up their rosters. That wouldn't have mattered except that Mark and I couldn't reach Pat.

I didn't have his cell phone at that time, so I was calling his office. I finally left a message and said, "I'm coming to Miami."

But it didn't matter what I said or wanted to do, I needed a contract offer from the Heat and I didn't have one. In the meantime, the Phoenix Suns were calling Mark offering me a roster spot with them. The Suns had a lot of what the Heat could offer—a warm-weather city, a team that had just gone to the conference finals the year before, and a coach in Mike D'Antoni who thought I would do well in his system. The chance to play with point guard Steve Nash was very attractive. My old Blazers teammate Jim Jackson was there, too. Not knowing how much time I had left, I wanted to play for a team that I thought could win a championship and the Suns were certainly one of them. They were also the only one interested in my services.

After about five days of not hearing from Riley, I told Mark to accept the Suns' offer. I officially signed it on August 18. Pat called me that morning. He had been on vacation in Italy. I guess there's one time in the year where he goes away and disconnects with everybody for a couple of days. When he left he knew I was being amnestied and figured, "Well, Brian's coming," so there was no reason to get something done right away. If he had called at any point and said, "You're signing with us. I'll talk to you when I get back from Italy," I would've told Mark to shut everything else down. That's all I would've needed. But I didn't know why Pat hadn't called and could only come to one conclusion—he was no longer interested. Considering how late

I became available and after the season I'd had with the Lakers, it certainly would've made sense.

But not to Pat.

"What're you doing?" he asked. "I thought we always agreed there'd be a place for you. You have a spot on this team. Here's what you do. You tell them that you're not going through with the thing."

"Coach. I gave them my word. I'm a man of my word. I can't break my word."

"I just always thought you knew you had a place here."

"But you weren't calling me back."

"I was in Italy. I didn't know." He got quiet for a moment and then said, "But you know what? They probably need you more than we do. I just wanted you to be on this team because we've got a chance to win one and I want you to win a championship."

The Heat, of course, did win a championship that year. Twenty-one games into the season, Pat came to coach the team. Do I ever think about how close I came to catching a ring? Yeah, yeah, I do. All the time. It wouldn't be the last time I just missed catching one, either.

If missing out on rejoining the Heat wasn't bad enough, I found out that the Phoenix Suns were signing another center and introducing us at the same press conference. "You guys will be sharing a car with the Burkes to the press conference," a Suns official told me.

"Which one?"

"Pat Burke."

"Oh," I said.

Of all the people they could have signed and introduced with me, it had to be Pat. See, we had some history. He was the starting center for the Orlando Magic during the 2002–03 season. The Magic beat us all four times we met that season, including a game in Miami where Pat threw the ball up over his head to beat the shot clock. The ball banked in off the backboard and the crowd—our crowd, small as it was—went crazy. I was not impressed. In fact, I was mad because I knew Riley would be on my ass for letting it happen.

After the game, a reporter asked how I felt about losing to the Magic. My mind was still on that stupid shot Pat took. "Well, you know things aren't going well for you," I said, "when Pat Who? throws it up over his head and it goes in."

I heard through the grapevine that Pat saw what I said in the newspaper, but he left the NBA to play in Europe the next few seasons so we never crossed paths again. Until the car ride in Phoenix.

Gina sat up front in the passenger seat, while I got in back with Pat and his wife, Peyton, who sat next to me. Gina knew the story about Pat and me, so she kept looking back to see what was happening. I could tell by Peyton's mannerisms she was waiting for something to happen, too.

Finally, Pat piped up, "Hey, you know what's funny? Remember when we played—"

I cut him off. "Yeah, I remember."

"I just wanted to bring that up, because it was so funny when they said that you said, 'Pat Who?'"

"Yeah, I said it. I said it because you threw up some bullshit over your head and made it."

"Well, I mean, it did go in. I was just so excited because I couldn't believe I had a decent game against Brian Grant. Because, you know, you're *Brian Grant*."

"Well, that was still some bullshit. But you know what? I apologize. Ladies, you heard me, right? I apologized."

Peyton turned to Pat and said, "See, I told you he was a good guy."

We became real tight after that. D'Antoni had recruited both of us, but after we got there he warned the whole team that he only played six or seven guys and while those guys would love him, the other six or seven would hate him. Pat and I probably thought we both would be among the six or seven playing—as I'm sure every player did. D'Antoni went with a deeper rotation the first couple of weeks to figure out who should be in his shorter one, so I actually got some time in eight of our first 11 games. Then my right knee locked up on me and I had to have surgery. I didn't play again until March.

It's not as if I had high expectations after I came in and played some pick-up games against the Suns' up-and-coming power forward Amar'e Stoudemire. He must've dunked on me at least five times that first day. There was a play where he got the ball and I thought, *He's not going to take off from that far out...*" Sure enough, he did. And crushed it. I was ready to quit the team. He remains, easily, as one of the most athletic guys I ever played with or against.

I didn't quit, but to keep ourselves connected to the team and feel like we had some value, Pat and I became scouts when we were on the road. The other guys knew we'd be hanging out somewhere since we weren't playing and would call us to get a report.

"How is it?" they'd ask.

"It's manageable," I'd say. "There's not a lot of people here, so people aren't going to be bothering you." They'd come out for a bit, but they couldn't hang as long as we did because they were going to have to play the next day. Pat being Irish, we seemed to wind up in a lot of pubs drinking Guinness, something I drank only because of him. More often than not, our teammates would roll back to the hotel while we'd look at each other and say, "Ah, might as well have another one."

The morning practice before any night game is called a shootaround. There was one road game where I noticed Pat getting up extra shots and just being generally more active than usual. "What are you getting ready for?" I asked.

"I feel like I might get a chance to play," he said.

He wouldn't come right out and say it, but apparently D'Antoni had pulled him aside and said, "Hey, we're going to need you tonight, so be ready. Okay?"

"Yeah, sure," Pat told him. But he never got in the game.

I didn't find out about all that until a day or so later, when we were walking off the court after the morning shootaround for our next game. D'Antoni came up to me and said, "We're probably going to play you tonight. Are you going to be ready?"

"Yeah, I'll be ready," I told him.

Pat waited until Mike had walked around the corner and then sidled up next to me. "Did D'Antoni just tell you to be ready because he's going to play you?"

"Yeah," I said.

"He told me the same shit last game."

"I don't know, Pat, I think he's going to play me."

I didn't play a minute.

In other ways, though, D'Antoni was alright. I was in so much pain a lot of the time that before he put me in at garbage time, he'd ask me if I wanted to go in or not. Most of the time I said yes. I'd had to let go of a lot of my pride at that point.

My Suns teammates could not have been more cool. My first eight or nine years in the league I had been on plenty of teams that had that one veteran who was there not to play but mostly just to practice and help the young guys get better or show them a few tricks to playing in the league. A few of those vets used to be able to ball but really couldn't anymore because they were physically broken down and sometimes they didn't get a whole lot of respect. There'd be some laughing at the old man on the team behind his back. It ticked me off. I appreciated the Suns because they didn't do that. Steve Nash, Raja Bell, and Shawn Marion set the tone and sent me out the right way. They told me, "We know what you used to be able to do. If you've got something to say, say it."

They even gave me a nickname: Ol' Jizzle. I don't know if it was Pat or Steve, but we were out getting something to eat and one of them said, "There goes ol' Jizzle." I'm not even sure what it meant, but I knew they liked me, so I rolled with it.

That made the situation easier on me because I'd seen the older cats who did get disrespected feel like they needed to snap back and talk some trash. It usually went something like, "If this was 10 years ago, I'd whup your young butt," which would lead to some younger player saying, "Yeah, but it ain't 10 years ago, so..." It made for a bad team atmosphere.

Kurt Thomas and I kept each other sharp earlier in the season, two old heads playing one-on-one after practice. We were both 33, the oldest on the team, but he got steady minutes until he suffered a stress fracture in his right foot in February and basically missed the rest of the season.

It was in one of those sessions that I now realize the disease let me know for the first time what it could do to me. This was the time I told you about earlier, when my leg simply refused to do what it had done my whole life. I blew by Kurt and went to dunk the ball and missed ugly.

That's when I realized I couldn't jump off my left leg the way I once could. I'm right-side dominant except when I shoot—my strength comes from my left side. I went to the Suns' trainer, who suggested it was just Father Time catching up with me but he made an appointment with a neurologist. He looked at my medical chart with all my surgeries listed and said, "I suspect you're going to see a lot of that in different places, because you've been in the league so long. You've had a good run and you played hard and been beat up."

If I'd had anything left, there might've been a chance for me to contribute. Despite what Stoudemire did to me in those first pick-up games, he announced a couple of days into training camp that he needed knee surgery. He came back in March to play three games but then shut it down again for the rest of the season. He never quite regained that same crazy athleticism I got to experience firsthand, but we still had a pretty good squad with Nash, Marion, Boris Diaw, Tim Thomas, Leandro Barbosa, and Raja, making it to the Western Conference finals, where we lost to the Dallas Mavericks. I then watched as Pat and the Heat came back against the Mavericks to win the 2006 championship in six games.

The Suns did knock out the Lakers in the first round, coming back from being down 3–1 in the series to win 4–3. Even though I only played a total of five minutes, it felt good to be on the right side of an outcome with the Lakers for once. We then beat L.A.'s other team in the second round, the Clippers, and I made my last appearance on an NBA court. D'Antoni surprised me by subbing me in for Diaw midway through the first quarter of the third game of the series. I managed to foul Clippers forward Elton Brand and take two jumpers in less than two minutes, missing both. Boris came back in for me and I didn't see the floor again. Ever, as it turned out. My right knee locked up and I didn't even dress for the series with the Mavericks.

On the night of the 2006 NBA draft, the Suns traded me and their first-round pick, Rajon Rondo, to the Boston Celtics for a 2007 first-round pick. Their GM, Danny Ainge, asked if I could just come in and be a player-coach type. "We have veteran players who respect you," he said. "We think you could help us." If I could've run at all, I would have said yes, but despite the surgery, my right knee was bothering me so much I could barely get up and down the court. I was already struggling with being a shadow of my former athletic self. I didn't want to show up and have anyone look at me hobbling around and wonder why I was even there. The Celtics, of course, were on their way to that 2008 title. In hindsight, I wish I had taken them up on it.

Instead, I went back to Miami and went to the Heat's first game and watched them receive their rings and unfurl a championship banner from the American Airlines Arena rafters. I was happy for them, but I couldn't stop fidgeting in the stands. I wasn't ready to be a spectator. I left at halftime and went home to hide out, wondering about the persistent twitch on the inside of my left wrist, fighting with Gina about not wanting to see anyone or do anything, and generally feeling sorry for myself.

chapter 11
Kings Fall

The greatest regret of my life is screwing up my marriage to Gina. I knew what I had, I just didn't know how to take care of it. I had an arrogance, partially created by how good she made me feel about myself. I felt as if nothing could take her away from me but me—and that's exactly what happened. I can say this: I will love Gina Grant until the day I stop breathing. We fought like cats and dogs at times but she was my one true love and I messed it up. Anything she did to me, I did to her a hundred times over. It's not as if I got with every girl I could, I was just careless. I'd get a phone number, think I'd thrown it away, and Gina would find it in my pants pocket. That's in between having children with two other women during our relationship.

I knew I'd hurt her then, but when the tables were turned it really brought it home. That's why I'm happy for her now. She has moved on and remarried and her career has taken off. She only deserves the best and I didn't always give that to her. I can say that since Gina, I haven't cheated in any relationship I've had. I just wish I'd been able to learn the value of that sooner. While my early life taught me how to take on physical challenges, it didn't prepare me for emotional ones. Especially when it came to relationships. Almost all of mine with girls growing up were on the sly. It was an all-out, do-whatever-it-takes competition with my cousins in our little town just to have one. There was no honor among my cousins and me, either; you did or said whatever it took to get the girl. It's not something I'm proud of now, I just didn't know better back then.

I love everyone in my family—my uncles, aunts, everybody. Always have, always will. But they weren't exactly the best role models on how to build and maintain a healthy relationship, either.

My mom, Gigi, was 18 years old when I was born. My dad, Tommy, was 17. They were so young my Aunt Jackie and her husband tried to adopt me, but my mom refused. "Nah," she said. "I'm not giving up my baby."

That didn't change even after my dad got busted breaking into a hardware store with a couple of buddies. The judge told them: "You've got two choices. Go to jail for a couple of years or join the Marines." They all chose the Marines. But when my dad went off to boot camp, my mom had no choice but to move in with her in-laws. Being a young mom, she got a lot of advice and it made things rough. It didn't take long for her to decide she'd rather move around the country and be a military wife than have her in-laws telling her all the things she was doing wrong as a mother.

At first, my dad was stationed at the Southern California Marine Corps base, Camp Pendleton, but we weren't there long and I was too young to remember anything about it. My first memories are from our next stop, Camp LeJeune, in Jacksonville, North Carolina. That's where my life-long fear of snakes began. We lived in a mobile home park and it was my third birthday. Our neighbor had a boa constrictor. I was scared just knowing an animal like that lived next door, but on my birthday the neighbor brought it out and tried to hand it to me, as if holding that big ol' snake was my birthday present. "Here, Brian, let it on you," he said. I'm sure I screamed. I can guarantee you I did not let it on me.

We went back and forth between Ohio and North Carolina a lot. We were poor, so that meant driving through the Appalachians in our beat-up green station wagon. Those mountains seemed so high, the trip seemed to take forever and the radiator always seemed to be overheating. We'd end up using all our water going uphill, which meant my dad had to put the wagon in neutral and coast on the downhill part until we could get more water. Sometimes my grandparents on my mom's side would come and get me and I'd live with them for a month or so, but the trip was just as long riding with them. I hated it.

After my dad got discharged, we moved back to Ohio, living in a house in Ripley for a while before moving to Grant Avenue in Georgetown. Before my dad died, he became my best friend and I came to love him as a father, but he wasn't ready to be either back then. I didn't think he was shit. A lot of my cousins felt the same way about their fathers. You can put some of that on us, the sons. We didn't realize what it was like trying to be a man back then, being Black and poor and living in the country. I can see now how hard it had to have been.

One thing my dad had going for him was that he was a really good-lookin' dude and the ladies loved him. I came home with my mom one time and my dad had a chick in the house. My mom went at them and my dad said, "You touch her, I'm gonna touch *you* up."

My mom didn't know what to do so she ran up the hill with me to her grandparents' house. She walked in crying and sat down.

"What the fuck is wrong with you, Gigi?" my grandmother asked.

"He's got her in the house!" my mom wailed.

"Well, you better get your ass down there and get her out," my grandmother said.

"If I do, he's going to come after my ass!"

"Well, shit!" My grandmother stood up and ran out the front door.

My grandfather yelled, "Hold on, Lizzy!" as he struggled to get on his boots. "Bean Butt," he said, looking at me, "you stay right there!"

I did until I heard someone screaming, "Help! Agghh!" I ran down the hill, where a group of about 30 people had gathered at the bottom, watching my grandmother slap the shit out of my dad's side chick.

Uncle John made a move to break it up, but his dad, my grandfather, Tom, warned him, "Boy, don't you ever put your hands on your mother. Back up!" Then he turned to Lizzy. "Damn, girl!" he said and cheered her on. "Alright! Alright!"

Grandma Lizzy was laying on top of the girl, exhausted. "Get her off me!" the girl said.

"Damn it," Lizzy said, "I can't hit you no more." That's when she bit the girl in the back and got her nickname, "Bite-her-in-the-back Lizzy." Bit her more than once, too, before my grandpa finally went over and helped her up.

Apparently, my grandmother had gone into my parents' house and dragged the chick out into the street. The chick pressed charges and we had to go to court. I didn't go but my mom did and gave me the details later. My grandmother walked into the court room first and then the side chick girl came in next. She still looked beat up. The judge introduced the case and then asked for the two of them to approach the bench.

We thought for sure Grandma Lizzy was going to jail. But the judge, a woman, said to the side chick, "If I ever see you in my courtroom for messing with a married man again, I'm going to put you in jail. Case dismissed."

There was a lot of that kind of dysfunction in my family growing up. My dad, Tommy, had four children outside of his marriage to my mom. My cousins and I were constantly fighting over attempts to steal each other's girlfriends. The worst fights I ever saw involved family members, hands down. It wasn't just a male thing, either. It could be sister vs. sister, aunt vs. uncle, you name it. And a lot of the beefs were about infidelity. As much as I never intended to follow in those footsteps, I sometimes wonder if I inherited some trait that led to my difficulties developing and nurturing a healthy relationship. Especially if there was alcohol involved. Drink enough, I learned, and values became situational—or to paraphrase the comedian Chris Rock, I became "as faithful as my options."

During my last year playing in Phoenix, Gina became involved in a dance exercise program called Zumba and quickly became one of their best instructors. That wasn't a surprise because she was so good-looking and she'd been dancing since she was a kid. But one of the program directors had messed around with the wife of a friend of mine and it didn't take long for me to suspect he might be going after Gina. I made those suspicions known to Gina, basically accusing her of cheating on me, calling her all kinds of names for it, and resenting that she was spending so much on her Zumba career.

I knew, deep down, that I should have supported her. She had done so many little things for me during my career. If I went on a road trip, I'd open my shaving kit and find a note from her thanking me for all I did for the family and being her "shining star." She understood how much stress came with being a professional athlete and fighting every practice and every game to keep your spot, and she would do whatever she could to make life easy for me away from the court. She also allowed me to make all the decisions, deferring to me because I was the big bread winner. I was used to feeling as if I ran the show and now that was changing. I was good with her pursuing her own thing, but I was stuck feeling depressed over my career ending and couldn't find my way past that to support her the way I should have.

Depression wasn't the only thing putting me in a fog. All of my surgeries had left me with bottles of Vicodin and Percocet. They definitely helped with the pain, but I found out they worked pretty well when I didn't have any pain, either. I made the excuse that my body was healing from all those years of beating it up and that I'd earned the right to do whatever I wanted. That's how it started.

It wasn't as if I walked into a doctor's office, said I was in pain, and asked if he could prescribe me something. I fell in the rabbit hole much more casually than that. I had a friend who, it turned out, could get me whatever I wanted. I don't think I ever came right out and asked him to get me anything; I just complained about how I'd been taking opioids and was running out and he said, "Oh, I can get those for you."

And I said, "Okay."

Once I had a steady supply, that's when my usage really ramped up. I crossed a threshold where the pills were not working anymore but I felt really shitty when I didn't take them. If I stopped for a couple of days I went through withdrawals, only I didn't know that's what was happening. My whole body would just seize up. We're not just talking about Vicodin; I started taking Oxycontin, too—Oxy 80s, the strongest ones they make.

At first I'd just buy a half dozen or so pills, but then I worked up to going through five or six in a two-day span. When they stopped working, I thought, "I have to get off this stuff." So I'd convince myself that I needed to buy them in bulk because I wanted to quit but I needed to wean myself off. That's how an addict's mind works. I was always making an excuse as to why I needed to keep going. Having the excuse that my knees were legitimately all messed up was a good one. (I conveniently ignored that there were a lot of people with messed-up knees who weren't poppin' pills.) If I didn't have any pills, well, I'd just have to be resourceful and do a couple of lines of cocaine instead. Only in an emergency, though—I wasn't a drug addict, I was just a former pro athlete who'd had more than a dozen surgeries and needed a little something to take the edge off. That's what I told myself.

Gina sensed something was wrong with me beyond being depressed about my NBA career being over. Around my first Christmas in retirement, she pushed me to seek professional help, but I didn't want to hear it. By spring, I finally was ready. In hindsight, so was Gina—to get away from me.

Philippe, as one of the first people I let back into the house, was one of the first to notice it. Gina asked if she could do something, I said she couldn't (of course, because I was an asshole) and she said, "Well, I'm going to do it anyway."

Philippe noticed the change in Gina's attitude toward me. After she left the room, Philippe said, "Brother, you need to get on top of that shit."

"Philippe, she's going to do what she's going to do," I said. Once I pulled out of my depression and we started being social as a couple again, we hit the clubs a few times.

Raphael Saddiq came out to visit. He knew how jealous I could be if any dude showed Gina any sort of attention, so when he saw Gina on the dance floor without me, he said, "She done lost her goddamn mind dancing like that."

"She's a great dancer," I said. "Let her have her fun."

Raphael looked at me with his eyebrows raised. "You sure have come a long way," he said.

He was right. There was a time if she went to the bathroom I'd watch her like a hawk all the way there and back. But it wasn't as if she was dirty dancing with dudes. She'd be out there with her girlfriends, a few dudes would try to dance with them, but in between songs she'd come over and sit next to me and then go back out on the floor. We weren't lovey-dovey or anything, but she never tried to embarrass me. I had put her through so much I couldn't begrudge her having a good time.

Besides, she had always been strong-willed; the difference was, there was a time when that will was dedicated to doing what was best for us. Now it seemed she was committed to doing what was best for her. I knew, deep down, that I'd forced that change of heart. Venting about how I thought she was doing me wrong was one thing, but I'd lost my privileges to tell her what she should do.

What I did next is called "doing a geographic" in recovery rooms. I convinced Gina that we should move back to Portland. I figured it would put some distance between her and the Zumba dude and me and the pills and that might, just might, give Gina and me a chance to come together again.

I found out pretty quickly Gina moved for the sake of the family, not me. She was gone roughly three weeks out of every month, traveling all over the world for Zumba—China, Rio,

Chile, France. It gave me a lot of time with our kids, but I was sure now she was having an affair. When she said she was going to Chile and didn't invite me, I said, "Fine. I'm going to Costa Rica to surf." I didn't talk to her for a few days and then called and cussed her out for giving up on us. There were so many times I could've turned the other way, taken it on the chin, accepted that she was messing around, suggested we get counseling, and tried to repair the damage. But I was too busy being hurt and feeling betrayed.

I'm sure Gina was thinking, *I forgave you for all you did. I raised your kids from other mothers. I kept the house together. You're depressed, you can't live with yourself, and I gave into an impulse—and now you can't forgive* me? I couldn't see that all back then the way I can now.

If I had the decision to do over again, I would not have filed for divorce. I would've hung in there for however long it took, stayed married, and hoped for a little bit of brightness to shine on her that changed her mind. I wish I had told myself, *Okay, you're hurt. Deal with it.* But I wasn't thinking that way. I didn't want our marriage to end, but I couldn't get past my ego. My last-ditch effort to save our marriage consisted of putting together a video of us that first summer in Jamaica for her birthday. I used Joe Cocker's "You Are So Beautiful" and one of my favorite songs by Sade, "I Couldn't Love You More," as the soundtrack. When we first got together, I played Sade all the time, especially that song. Her mom printed out the lyrics and gave them to Gina. She, in turn, took the sheet with a rose from a bouquet I gave her and put them together in a frame.

I got all the kids together and brought Gina in, said, "I made this for you," and played the video.

After it was over, Gina said, "That's nice," and walked out. That's when I knew it was over.

After I filed for divorce, I moved into a second house and that's when my drug use really took off. I went to a men's Bible study, hoping to find some answers, and that's where someone mentioned Alcoholics Anonymous and handed me the AA Big Book, but I said, "Nah, I don't need that."

But the shackles were off now. When I was living with Gina, I had to hide what I was doing because she could always tell when I was high. Now there was no one around to stop me and if someone came by, it didn't matter who they were—Jermaine, Brian Berger—I wouldn't answer the door. If I couldn't find pills, I took whatever I could get my hands on.

The coke drove me over the edge because coming down from it will depress a normal person. For someone dealing with the depression induced by Parkinson's, adding the downer of cocaine withdrawal made that black hole the next day seem bottomless.

I finally came to one morning, alone, staggered into the bathroom, looked at myself in the mirror, and started crying.

How did it come to this? I'd blamed Parkinson's. I'd blamed my ex-wife. I'd blamed everybody but myself for the state of my life. I finally stared into that mirror and said. "You did this to you. They didn't do this. You did."

I spent an hour looking into that mirror, sobbing, when I was reminded of a conversation I'd had with a friend, another ex-NBA player. He had talked about substance abuse and the problem he'd once had. I called him up. He asked for my address and came right over.

I answered the door. I knew how ratty I looked and smelled. I was embarrassed but he didn't care. He gave me a big hug and said, "I've talked to someone and I want you to talk to them."

It was a woman who handled the in-take service for a recovery center in Tucson, Arizona. I was in a daze. This was moving really fast.

"We have a bed waiting for you whenever you can get here," she said.

"He'll be there tonight," my friend said.

"I don't think there are any flights," I said.

Takes one to know one. He wasn't going to let me wiggle out of this. "He'll be there first thing in the morning." He stayed and we talked. He shared a few of his experiences and I told him a little about what I had been doing. I cried some more and then made some phone calls to let people know what I was about to do.

It's funny how I thought I had everyone fooled by staying locked away inside my house. "I know you don't know this, but I kind of have a problem with—"

They'd cut me off. "You're going to treatment? Thank God."

"Damn. You knew?"

"Everybody knows, B. We were scared for you. With the pain pills and whatever else. People are dying from that stuff."

"I guess I'm making the right decision then."

I wasn't 100 percent sure of that. I was terrified of how Gina might react. I feared she would take the kids from me, more than anything. She started crying when I told her. "I am *so* happy for you," she said through the tears. "I know this has been tough for you, but just know, even if we're not together, I will *always* have your back."

That helped me go through with the trip to Tucson. Amanda and Monica were supportive, too. "Do what you have to do," Amanda said. I got the support I needed from everyone.

It was still hard to get on the plane. I ended up taking an afternoon flight. My buddy drove me. He stood there and watched me walk into the airport and through security. I could feel him watching and that was enough to get me onto the plane.

A guy from the recovery center met me at the Tucson airport. I found out later a lot of people checking in figured it was their last chance to get smashed so they really went at it. I assumed I'd be in trouble if I showed up high or drunk, so I was completely sober and nervous as hell, wondering what I had got myself into. The driver picked up on all that.

"I know you're scared," he said. "Don't be. You're in the right place. If you let your Higher Power work for you, it'll work for you. If you don't put anything into it, you won't get anything out of it."

My biggest fear was being recognized and outed. I imagined the scroll on the bottom of the TV: "Brian Grant has entered a drug rehabilitation center...."

After a couple of days, I realized that I was simply with a bunch of addicts and alcoholics trying to find a solution to their problem, counselors included. They didn't really care who you were. Trying to recover from a fucked-up life was a great equalizer.

The only thing I hated about the place were the snakes. I know some people go through withdrawals and have hallucinations that often include imaginary snakes, but these were real ones and I was jumping over them every day. Black snakes and rattlesnakes. We walked out of a meeting one day and someone said, "Brian, look down." There was one right at my feet. I took off on a sprint, bad knees and all.

It was a relief to hear other people's stories. I had come to believe I was the worst person in the world and no one could be as fucked up as I felt, but after hearing what other people had been through I felt something I hadn't felt in a long time: I was thankful.

My kids called and told me, "We love you, dad, we're so proud of you." Gina said the same.

After I got out, I was told to attend 90 recovery meetings in 90 days and find a sponsor, someone who would take me through the 12 Steps of recovery and keep me connected to the program. Being back in Portland, I still struggled with the idea of being outed. Any time I walked into a meeting I could feel the eyes on me and the instant recognition.

I was completely sober for nine months. I did my 90 in 90 but I didn't get a sponsor. The paranoia of being outed led me to scale back to a couple of meetings a week. There are hundreds of them in the Portland area, but I'd only go to one particular one where I knew everybody.

It didn't take long for the idea to pop in my head, "Alcohol wasn't my issue. Pain pills were. I'm allowed to have a beer." I shared that in a meeting and had six old heads come up to me afterward. "C'mon, let's talk a little bit about what you shared today," one of them said. "It's real easy to think what you're thinking. We've all been there. Alcohol might not have brought you in here, but if you really think about it, it's probably where it started." They gave me their phone numbers and told me if I needed a sponsor to call one of them.

I was feeling so good I didn't feel the need for meetings anymore. A few weeks went by and I decided to have that beer. It didn't take long for my brain to tell me, "C'mon, B, we're good, man, we can handle that shit."

I went looking for pills, found some, and started the whole vicious cycle over again. I know I disappointed everyone, all the people who were so happy and relieved I'd gone into rehab, all the people who stood by me. Somehow I failed to think about any of them once I started to think about that one beer.

To complicate matters even more, I decided to get married again.

During my stretch of sobriety, I had accepted my Parkinson's diagnosis and decided to shift the focus of my foundation from helping terminally ill kids like Woody, Dash, and Jovita to supporting those with PD. That gave me the chance to meet Michael J. Fox and attend one of his fundraisers in New York City. It was packed with famous people from the entertainment industry: movie director Martin Scorsese, actor Ryan Reynolds, and Roger Daltrey, the lead singer of The Who, to name a few. Millions of dollars were donated to fund research for a cure.

Michael thought I could be a big help if I used my celebrity and connections to bring awareness to the disease, but he was pretty blunt with me about what it took to do that.

"You've got to give up your vanity, man," he said. "You're going to be standing up in front of people talking and your arm is going to start shaking or your foot jiggling and you've got to be okay with that. It's not for everybody and if it's not for you, that's okay. Because once you step into that arena, you're in it. There's no stepping in and stepping out."

The suggestion that I might not be capable of something triggered a familiar feeling—the desire to prove him wrong.

He was right, though—it wasn't easy. After years of hearing kids and adults alike say, "Look, there's Brian Grant!" I had to get comfortable with a kid looking at me and asking, "What's wrong with that man, mommy?" It doesn't help that when I'm nervous, it makes my tremors and twitches become even more noticeable.

But another part of my competitive nature kicked in after I went to his fundraiser. With Michael being an actor and the room full of people in the entertainment industry, I expected something a little more exciting. The speakers were reading off a teleprompter and there was no entertainment. But I couldn't argue with the results and Michael clearly knew what he was doing, because they raised $4 million. My situation in Portland, though, was completely different. I wasn't a movie star and I couldn't fill a room with that many deep pockets. I felt like I had to do something to get people in Portland excited about the cause. When I got back to discuss doing an event, I said, "If we're going to do something and it's like that, then I don't want to do it." I took a page out of Pat Riley's book—if I was going to ask people to donate their time and money to Parkinson's research, I had to be ready to give them something memorable in return, something that made them feel whatever they did was worth it. Pat figured into making that a reality.

Nothing was bigger in Portland than the Rose Garden, and that's where we decided to hold our event. The idea of having a formal catered dinner, auction, and live entertainment on the arena floor got everyone excited. We came up with a list of entertainers that we knew or had recently seen that had blown us away, and that had some sort of connection to Portland, basketball, or both.

My friend Raphael Saddiq agreed to do a set. My cousin Jermaine knew comedian and movie actor Gary Owen had hosted several comedy specials for Shaquille O'Neal and suggested we get him to do his stand-up act. I had seen a group perform at New Year's Eve in Portland called the MarchFourth Marching Band—it was like a musical version of Cirque du Soleil. They have horn and percussion sections, along with some electric guitars and they play while stilt walkers and acrobats and jugglers perform. We called the whole thing the "Shake It 'Til We Make It Gala." There was a red carpet for all the celebrities to do interviews as soon as they arrived in the arena and hosts and hostesses to guide everyone to their tables.

We were able to put it all together. I don't know that Portland had seen anything quite like it before or since. We did a countdown and then the stilt walkers, followed by the marching band, appeared from behind big, red curtains. It felt like a mix between an African tribal dance and Mardi Gras. Instant party mode. My friends from the basketball world and beyond flew in from everywhere to be a part of it—Charles Barkley, Bill Russell, and many of my old teammates from both Miami and Portland. Muhammad Ali and Michael J. Fox, as fellow PD sufferers, came as well. The gala included a golf tournament the next day and Michael had everyone laughing when he joked, "It's a Parkinson's fundraiser, and you have a putting contest?" he began. "Who's the sick mind who thought of that?" He then gave the entire audience a chilling sense of what it's like to be diagnosed with PD.

"You're in the middle of the road with your feet stuck in a bucket of cement and you can hear a bus coming," he said. "You can't see it, but the roar tells you it's steadily getting closer. You just don't know when it's going to arrive."

I also used my "forever" card with Pat and asked him to be one of the speakers. The only mistake I made was in agreeing to speak right after him. Pat told a story about going whitewater rafting and how the instructor told him that everyone at some point, no matter what they did, would find themselves tossed into the river and that they would then "have to participate in their own rescue and find their way back to the boat."

He then related it to me and my battle with Parkinson's and helping others who were doing the same. "Brian," he said, "is participating in his own rescue. He's swimming back to the boat."

He then played a video he had made with clips from all the big moments of my playing days set to Rascal Flatts' song, "My Wish." The lyrics had the whole place getting choked up:

"My wish, for you, is that this life becomes all that you want it to,

Your dreams stay big, your worries stay small,

You never need to carry more than you can hold,

And while you're out there getting where you're getting to,

I hope you know somebody loves you, and wants the same things
too,

Yeah, this, is my wish."

I looked over at the table of Blazers' officials and mouthed, "Why didn't we think of a video?"

Pat still wasn't done. Before he left the stage, he announced that the Miami Heat were donating $25,000. "We love you, Brian," he said and started to walk off. Then he turned back to the microphone and added, "Oh, and one more thing—me and my wife, Chris, we're going to match that with $25,000 of our own."

That's my coach, I thought.

The live auction came next. Karl Malone, my old Jazz nemesis, contributed a once-in-a-lifetime item by making good on my suggestion that I hoped one day we could go fishing together: the chance to go on an Alaskan fishing trip with me and him. It was so popular that in the middle of the auction he agreed to do a second trip.

(Funny moment from that trip: Karl and I had a chance to talk about our battles on the court while we were up there. "Even as a young guy, I really respected that you left it on the court," he said. "Some guys want to fight in the tunnel or take it somewhere else.")

My foundation work for Parkinson's also provided the forum for me to eventually patch up my relationship with Tommy, my dad. The days I resented him for cheating on my mom and treating me bad just because I'd grown taller than him were behind us. I'd come to understand that if I had been in his shoes, I might've reacted the same way—in some ways, I did react the same way, as far as being unfaithful. If I was okay with who I had become as a man, I had to be okay with him—because he'd had a part in making me that man.

I can't remember which subsequent gala it was, but *Sports Illustrated* had just done a story on me and my battle with Parkinson's. We had placed an issue of the magazine on every table. In it, the dark side of my relationship with my dad had been included but not its current state. It also didn't include Amani as one of my children. As part of my speech, I corrected those oversights and spoke directly to my dad in front of everyone. "You're my best friend and I love you," I said.

I was on my way to the after-party at the Nines Hotel when my cell rang. It was Michael. My head was still buzzing from the fact that so many dignitaries had showed up and that my city of Portland had showed out. And now I had Michael J. Fox hitting my cell phone like we were boys. "Hey, what's up, man?" I said.

"Are you going to the after-party?" he asked.

"Yeah, I'm going to be there in a little bit."

"Alright. I'm going to meet you up there."

Katrina, a rep from his Foundation, told me later, "He never goes to after-parties. Ever." I found myself at a table with Michael, Pat, and Raphael.

"Hey, thank you for this," Michael said. "This was incredible. I expected big things, but this was crazy. You're actually making me think about the way we do things."

It was more than the fact that we were able to donate $350,000 to his foundation. He had The Roots performing at his next fundraiser and big screens everywhere with various artistic video content playing on them, with a Jamaican theme running through all of it. I felt very flattered. Our event had clearly made an impression. Don't let anybody tell you Marty McFly isn't competitive, either.

Allison Castelli, who worked for my agent, Mark, was one of the reasons for our success. When we started working on the event, Mark suggested she handle all the marketing for it. We were happy to get the help. On our first conference call, they didn't hear me join and so I heard someone warn Allison that I "like to drop a lot of F bombs."

I couldn't help letting them know I was on the line by saying, "Hey, what the fuck do you guys want?"

Allison worked remotely from Chicago the entire time, but we wanted her to enjoy the gala with us. When her mother died a few weeks beforehand, we told her we'd understand if she didn't make it, but we'd still like to fly her out. She took us up on the offer. Everybody had the same reaction when they finally saw her: "Ohhh, so *that's* Allison."

I liked working with her and, like everybody else, thought she was stunningly attractive, but I was working really hard on being a different person. I had been reflecting on all the bad shit I had done in my life and where that had come from. What is it about me that made me act and think the way I did? How do I change?

The old me would've pursued Allison right off the bat without a second thought. The new me decided I should focus on the foundation and, since we had a working relationship, keep it strictly professional.

My kids were the ones who helped flip all that. Allison decided to relocate to Portland. Creating an encore to the first gala and refining how I could best serve the Parkinson's community required all of us working closely together, so it made sense. With Gina traveling a lot, our four kids—Elijah,

Jaydon, Anaya, Maliah—were my responsibility. They fell in love with Allison before I did. They were always talking about funny moments they'd had with her or things she'd done for them. The turning point came when I decided to take the kids up to the cabin and asked Allison if she wanted to come with us. I swear my primary motive was to make the kids happy by having her there. I was still moping a lot because of everything going on with Gina, but the first day out on the boat, everyone kept whispering to me about how great Allison was.

On the drive back to Portland, Allison and I talked. I told her I wasn't sure what to do with our relationship, but that I liked being her friend and I didn't want to mess it up.

We kept it platonic until Sade came to town and I took Allison to the concert. It was on after that, but I still was committed to being above board, so I told her either we had to stop messing around or she had to stop working for the foundation. She quit.

It was a mistake, and it was all my doing. Allison is a great woman, but I was looking for someone to help me raise my daughters and fill the void Gina had left. As I see it, I jumped head-first into a pool, not realizing it was empty.

My commitment to doing the right thing didn't include staying completely sober, either. I was slipping off the beam. I had stopped going to recovery meetings and I'd have a few beers or a glass of wine now and then. I was honest with Allison, in that I told her I'd been through rehab; I just wasn't doing any of the things someone who has been through rehab does to keep from going to rehab again. I thought marrying Allison could fix my life, if not me. The kids—my girls, especially—needed someone who could do their hair and talk about feminine subjects better than I could. (I had always relied on Gina for that.) I took my best shot at doing my daughters' hair for them, but I wasn't very good at it. There were mornings they went to school not exactly looking tip-top.

After a year of dating, Allison and I went to the Justice of the Peace in Portland, got married, and had our first child, Brian, or "BB," as we like to call him.

It only took a couple of months into the marriage before I convinced myself I could fortify the beer or the wine with a pill now and then. I started pulling away from Allison. One day she walked in and said, "Brian, I know you're high right now."

I acted offended. "What are you talking about? I've been sitting here watching TV."

She was on to me the same way Gina had been. If I spent all day watching someone fish on TV, it was a dead giveaway. "Every time you get high, you come in and put on the same channel and I have to sit here and watch you nod off," she said.

I was caught. I didn't care. "Okay, and?"

"You need to get help."

"I already had help. I don't need help."

It went another month or so like that and then one day I came home and my girls weren't there. Allison left a note to call her. "Where are Anaya and Maliah?" I asked when I got her on the phone.

"You have to call Gina," Allison said.

I did. Allison wasn't the only one on to me. "Brian, you're struggling again and until you get help the girls won't be coming over," Gina said. "I'm not going to stop the boys from coming over because they'll say, 'Forget you, mom, I'm going over to see dad to make sure he's alright.'"

She was right. It was as if Amani, Elijah, and Jaydon were the adults and I was the teenager they had to worry about.

"Dad, what are you doing?" Elijah asked one day. "You're going to kill yourself."

Allison went back to Chicago and took BB with her. That just left me and the boys. They would search the house looking for my stash and then flushing it down the toilet. They wouldn't tell me, they'd just do it. I'd find out when I went to take something and it was gone.

"Why did you do that? Do you know how much that shit cost?"

"Yeah, but you don't need that shit," Jaydon said.

"You're right," I'd say. And they were. But I was still helpless to stop.

There's a line in recovery about the point at which someone asks for help: being sick and tired of being sick and tired. I reached that point. Again. I called my foundation director, Charisse, and asked her to find me a rehab center in Oregon. Charisse wasn't surprised by the request—she'd known for a couple of months that I had been slipping. She found a Betty Ford clinic 30 minutes south of Portland, in Newberg. She sat with me as I broke down about the mess I'd made of my life again and drove me to the clinic.

However scared I might've been about running into someone I knew in Tucson, it didn't compare to going to Newberg. It wasn't even a question. Everybody knew who I was. They were very professional, but there's still that unmistakable moment of recognition. This time I needed to detox before I could enter the program. I was in detox for three days; I didn't need three days but I was afraid of joining the other inpatients. They finally sent one of them in to see me. "Just walk around," he said. "I guarantee you'll see this place is safe. I know who you are but I'm focused on dealing with my shit. We all are."

I took a walk around the grounds. The other inpatients were sitting around smoking cigarettes or dipping tobacco. "How you guys doing?" I asked but I didn't stop to talk.

The next day, I walked through again. I exchanged some brief chit-chat with a few people. What put me at ease was that no one was coming up to me. Well, one person did but all he said was, "It does a lot to see you in here. That's courage."

I didn't feel courageous; I felt grateful. "You guys are doing a lot for me," I said. "You're making me feel welcome. You're making me feel like I'm no different than anybody else."

I had to commit to staying 30 days without leaving. After that, you can stay for another 60 or 90 days but have a car and get permission to leave. I elected to stay another 60 days. "This is going well for me, but I need more," I told Allison. "I need time to figure out where I need to go. To feel safe enough, to trust myself enough, to get out."

"Of course," she said.

What helped a lot was sharing exactly what I'd done with the other inpatients. They'd tell me their stories and I'd tell them mine and it made me realize there was no difference between us. They were dealing with the same demons I had. By staying the extra 60 days, I also saw two or three guys leave and by the time I left they were back for another round, a little more beat up and a little more convinced they had to change how they were living.

While Allison supported me going to rehab, it strained our relationship. We had a second boy, Max, but I was a different person coming out than I had been going in. Allison has always been a great mom, but wanting my kids to have a mother wasn't enough of a reason to stay married. The divorce drove me to stay closer to people in the program. At least for a while. I still have lapses. I've managed to stay away from the pills, but any time my Parkinson's medication isn't working to reduce my tremors, I use the excuse that a beer or a glass of wine will do the trick. Which it does. But I also know there's a voice in my head patiently waiting for me to get bored or in some sort of emotional pain so it can whisper, "One pill won't hurt and, in fact, it might do you a lot of good. You can handle it, B. Look at all you're dealing with. Let it all go. The pill will let it all go...."

My friend Raphael Saddiq knows all too well what addiction can do. He recorded an entire album about it, titled *Jimmy Lee*, named after his older brother, a heroin addict who died of AIDS. There's a song on the album about me, too, called "Kings Fall."

"I wake up, I call the man
To see what's in the man's hands
He comes by and drops it off
To let me know how much the pills cost
(I want you to be my)
I disappoint myself sometimes
'Cause I can't stop my bottom line
My kids cry, my wife's scared
My friends think I'm better off dead (Be my)
My eyes roll and I'm scared
I find myself lyin' back in the bed
I'm hiding out, I keep the blinds closed
I could see witches flyin' everywhere (I want you to be my)

320

I could see witches flyin' everywhere (I want you to be my)
Where, where, where, where, where (I want you to be my)
The supplier, my provider, and all those things
(I want you to be my)
My provider, and supplier, and all those things, and all those
things
(I want you to be my)
Even when I'm clean
I'm still a dope fiend
Everyone is always trying tell me something
(I want you to be my)
I wake up, I feel things crawlin'
But nobody wants to see a strong man fallin'
(I want you to be my)
I used to be
Everybody's hero
Shakin' hands and kissing babies
(I want you to be my)
Wondering what to do, Lord."

I was flattered in a way to have a song written about me, even if it was about my struggle with opioids. He told me more than once: "Don't get down on yourself. We're all addicts. Some are addicts of sugar, some are addicts of liquor or pain killers. We've all got addictions. What we've got to do is stick together and work it out. Know that I'm always going to be there for you."

After the big gala and all the people like Raphael who made it such a huge success, I felt an obligation to keep it going, while also wondering how we'd be able to match, much less surpass it. But we had the eyes of the Parkinson's community on us and being a one-hit wonder wasn't going to cut it.

chapter 12

Climbing the Mountain

Throughout my playing career, setbacks and disappointment provided the fuel I needed to reach the next level. I don't know if I would've become the player I became if it had been different, if I had people telling me I was "all that" from the jump. But I never had to look very hard to find someone making it clear they didn't think I was shit. You don't think I can play because I only had one year of high school basketball at a small-town school in Ohio? Cool—I'll prove you wrong. You don't think I can ball at the college level because I was Xavier's last choice for a scholarship? Cool—I'll prove you wrong. You don't think I can make it in the NBA because I spent four years at a mid-major and you've never heard of me? Cool—I'll prove you wrong. You don't think I can compete as an undersized power forward against Karl Malone and other superstars at my position? Cool… you know the answer by now.

What made Parkinson's a different challenge is the depression that came with it, especially in those months when I didn't know I had the disease and the months after that when I refused to do anything about it. It sapped my energy and that had been my answer for every problem: work longer, work harder, work. I always had a reputation for being the first one in the gym and the last one out. Working hard wasn't a challenge, it was my solution. That's what was so confusing; now I found myself stuck to the couch or crawling back in bed. It was as if I'd been unplugged. I couldn't understand why. I realized how much my self-confidence came from being an athlete and in great shape. Now, not wanting to take my shirt off or look at myself in the mirror only added to the depression.

It helped once I finally accepted I had Parkinson's, but I refused to accept that it was different from any other challenge I had faced. I had defied what people predicted I could and couldn't do for most of my life, so why should I accept that I couldn't beat Parkinson's? At the very least, couldn't I battle the disease to a draw? Surely there was a pill or a procedure that could get rid of it; after all, pills and procedures had solved every other physical ailment I'd ever had. Medicine plus my willpower plus my pain threshold had been my formula for success. It allowed me to perform against the NBA's best, despite physical problems that would've put most people on the shelf. All I needed was that formula to work one more time for me. There must be a way… right, Doc?

Right, Doc?

Doc?

I've been dealing with Parkinson's for well over a decade now and what I've learned is how much we still don't know about it or the treatments for it. Dr. Nutt, for example, started by prescribing a standard medication called Azilect. It reduces the shaking and stiffness caused by the disease, but it also makes you lethargic, which wasn't going to help me with my struggles to work out and lose weight. The diet restrictions to avoid high blood pressure and a possible heart attack were truly depressing: no wine, no beer, no chocolate, no coffee, no hot dogs, no bacon—or any other meat you can imagine on a pizza—and no aged cheeses or cultured dairy products, so no traditional pizza, either. I couldn't have anything that had Tyramine in it.

Which is how I found out what most of the things I liked to eat and drink contained: Tyramine.

I lasted about a month before I started looking for an alternative.

That's how I found the Rising Health Wellness Center in Vancouver, Washington, not far from Portland. The center was run by Dr. Daniel Newman, a traditional doctor who, like Philippe, had also studied Chinese medicine and believed in the power of naturopathy, the philosophy of treating or preventing disease by relying on diet, exercise, and massage.

Dr. Newman, though, also believed in the power of conventional drugs, especially when it came to treating Parkinson's. He offered both methods to his patients.

Most people with PD choose a particular form of treatment. Not me. I was going to try everything. I still had it somewhere in the back of my mind that there was a formula to keep my Parkinson's in permanent remission, the same way I got a shoulder or knee fixed with the right combination of surgery, exercise, and medication. I just needed to find it.

Dr. Newman was a willing guide for my quest. He prescribed a long list of both drugs and natural supplements; I not only tracked down every single one of his but through research added a few of my own.

The problem, of course, is that it's hard to pinpoint what is actually working. It takes months of experimenting with different combinations and keeping detailed records of what was taken, what time of day and what the reaction was. Another problem is that it's hard to know if how you're feeling is the medication, something you ate or drank, your mood, or even the weather. Or some combination of all that.

I had the money, time, and desire to try everything and anything. Some studies suggest metals and minerals absorbed into the body are the problem, so I had the water coming into my house tested for arsenic and other impurities. I wondered if pesticides had anything to do with me getting PD, so I ate only organic foods. I learned that some personal hygiene products have metals in them, so I changed my deodorant, toothpaste, and soap to all-natural brands.

Dr. Newman could not have asked for a more willing guinea pig. He tested my blood every time I went to see him and drew all sorts of conclusions from the reports. They showed I was deficient in a lot of things that help to metabolize dopamine in the brain, so he put me on a regimen to replace all the elements I was missing. I got hooked up to IV bags of vitamin A and C. I took hypodermic shots of glutathione, a natural antioxidant that the brain produces to help leach heavy metals and poisons. I took something called 5-HTP, which breaks down into tyrosine, which then produces dopamine.

My body can do this, said the little voice in my head, *I just need to provide it with the right ingredients.*

Between training as an athlete, my surgeries, and working with Philippe, I thought I had a pretty good grasp of what makes the human anatomy work from the neck down, but now I found myself earning a degree in neuroscience as well. The brain, I learned, is protected by the blood brain barrier and I had one that didn't work very well. Glutathione is the key ingredient for a strong barrier and is measured in basic terms: plus-plus, plus, negative, or negative-negative. Dr. Newman diagnosed me as negative-negative, meaning a lot of bad stuff had easy access to my brain.

Gina no doubt would've said that only confirmed what she already knew.

If my blood tests showed I was off a minuscule amount of anything, Dr. Newman prescribed a supplement. The first time I sensed we were going overboard is when he screened my blood for Lyme disease and said I had that, too. Or at least he suspected I had it.

"How is it you're not sure?" I asked.

"Well, we took two tests," he said. "One showed you had it, and the other one showed you didn't. The more reliable one is the one that said you have it, so we'll just treat you as if you have it."

I convinced myself this program was working, but the whole process got expensive in a hurry. No wonder they were always so happy to see me at the Wellness Center pharmacy. They were always suggesting something new and I was always eager to try it. "You need a bottle of 5-HTP? We sell that. Or how about some tyrosine? It's listed right outside on the sign, only $95." I was spending close to $4,000 a month just on IVs and supplements.

That wasn't all. I was also taking four packets of traditional medicine prescribed by Dr. Newman four times a day. We're talking a combination of 20-plus supplements and pills in each packet.

I worked with Dr. Newman for nearly 18 months, but I lasted about four weeks on the take-everything-and-anything regimen. It got to the point that I dreaded walking into my game room, where I had turned the bar into my personal laboratory of pills, powders, herbs, vitamins, and cod-liver oil. One of the pills had these little beads in it and I swear I could hear them jiggle all the way down my throat. I started having stomach problems. I hate throwing up, but eventually all those pills were coming back up not long after I swallowed them. It got to where just thinking about having to take them would make my gag reflex fire.

I came to the conclusion that putting all those substances in my body couldn't be healthy, especially for my kidneys. For a moment, I could see the flaw in thinking more is better. Even good stuff can become bad stuff if there's too much of it.

My faith in Rising Health ran out around the same time. I felt as if they were taking advantage of my desperation to beat the odds instead of offering guidance. I don't remember them ever saying, "No, you don't need that." Maybe they saw me as an ATM or maybe they were as eager to find a solution as I was. All I know is no one else was coming in and filling their shopping basket the way I was. The recommendations were expensive and endless and, ultimately, not having the impact I had hoped.

Even after I stopped going to Rising Health, I was never short on people willing to sell me a cure. Once I publicly announced that I had the disease, all kinds of people approached me. A guy who worked at the Blazers' arena told me about his connection with a clinic in Mexico that could cure Parkinson's with a blood-cleansing method that simply hadn't been approved in the U.S. For $15,000, he would hook me up with them. The treatment, he said, would cost another $35,000. They supposedly had other people with PD who had tried it that you could call to hear their testimonials.

"It really works," he said. "You can be cured."

"That would be great," I said. "But what's the first $15,000 for?"

"I'll make sure you get with the right people and they take care of you," he said. "Isn't it worth your health?"

Translation: *I'm offering you a chance to live, dude—are you going to let money get in the way of finding out if it will work?*

As much as I believed that sometimes you had to take risks to get what you want—playing with a torn labrum, turning down a maximum-salary contract—I'd come across enough Slim Shadys that I could spot one. There were other procedures that promised to treat Parkinson's, usually found in foreign countries that weren't under the jurisdiction of the U.S. Food and Drug Administration (FDA). I read about surgeons in China who had developed a procedure where they planted stem cells in your brain, supposedly to regenerate the dopamine producers. The website was up front about the odds. Seven patients had undergone the procedure, it said. Three were a success; two didn't have any effect; and two were fatal.

I had enough sense to run that one past Dr. Nutt before I hopped on a plane. But this will tell you my level of desperation to find a cure and my willingness to believe I had special powers when it came to beating the odds. I thought long and hard about doing it. I even imagined myself telling people after the fact: "Sure, a couple people died—but I didn't!"

There were also a few times I considered keeping Dr. Nutt in the dark and just going for it. I found out later that all my friends, knowing my impulsive nature, were on alert not to let me make any abrupt trips to China or Mexico.

I'm sure anyone looking at the offers objectively could tell right away how fishy they were, but anyone diagnosed with PD is more inclined to wishful thinking than objectivity. Hoping and praying you can avoid what eventually happens to anyone who has Parkinson's puts you in a different headspace. I had former teammates—Kobe Bryant and Jermaine O'Neal, to name two—who had made trips to Europe to get successful treatment on their knees, treatment that hadn't been approved in the U.S. I tried to convince myself that this was the same kind of thing. If that worked for them—and they said it did—isn't it possible one of these rare (and expensive) treatments could work for me? Maybe they weren't all that well-known because they were expensive and most people couldn't afford them. These are the kind of conversations I had with myself every time I opened my laptop, typed "Parkinson's cures" in the search engine and made another discovery.

After I moved on from Rising Health and Dr. Newman, I tried a more traditional approach by taking a combination of drugs called Carbidopa-Levodopa, which both produces dopamine and expedites its delivery to the brain. Sounds like the perfect one-two punch, right? Neurologists are convinced now that anyone should use C-L right away, but when I was first diagnosed I got mixed messages. One neurologist told me, "You should get on it as quickly as possible," while another cautioned, "Wait until you really need it." The first approach is all about having the best quality of life now. That doctor also told me at the time, "You're what, 37 years old? You could hold off on meds until you're 42, but you're going to deal with symptoms every day that are going to get progressively worse. You should think about quality of life now instead of down the road."

I started off taking three doses of Carbidopa-Levodopa a day. Then I found some supplements that have allowed me to cut down to two doses. I've looked into a small fanny-pack-sized pump that you can hook up to a tube that feeds into your stomach; the location of the tube avoids the effect of your stomach acid on the drug, providing a lower, steadier dosage. I'm still weighing that one; my ego hasn't come to grips with having a tube permanently poking out of my abdomen just yet.

The downside is that the drug does not stop Parkinson's from killing the brain cells that produce dopamine, which means you have to keep increasing your dosage. Large doses of Carbidopa-Levodopa can then lead to a nasty little side effect called dyskinesia, which is a lot like the twitching and tremors caused by Parkinson's. But it's not. The head bobbing, body swaying, or maybe just an eye or hand twitching is a result of being over-medicated. Only the brain knows how to regulate the flow of dopamine a person needs from minute to minute; adding more through pills is flooding the system. It's hard for the average PD patient, at home, to know exactly how much of the drug is getting from their stomach to where it's needed, their brain, but chances are it's going to be too much or too little. When it's the wrong amount, your brain sends unintended signals and you end up with the wiggles and the twitches. My buddy, Ben Petrick, went through that for a while. He was diagnosed even younger than me, at 22, a couple of years into his career as a catcher for the Colorado Rockies. He kept it under wraps long enough to get five seasons in before he had to retire. He uses the pump now and it seems to be working for him.

Parkinson's symptoms can vary. A lot. Some people experience dystonia, a condition where a particular part of their body will freeze up, like your toes or eyes or forearm. There's also a brain glitch that causes your entire body to momentarily freeze, making it look as if they have suddenly turned to stone.

Nice, huh? The first time one of my PD-afflicted friends suddenly froze in the passenger seat of my car, I didn't know what was happening. When he came out of it and explained it to me, I thought to myself, *I want to avoid that shit at all costs.* Now you know why I opted not to go the C-L route in the first place and hoped, instead, to find a more holistic, natural kind of treatment.

I should've warned you: talking to someone with PD about their medication is like talking to a diehard golfer about his game—you're going to get excruciating detail about the endless search for the formula to an inexact science. That's because everyone who has PD is performing their own experiments on a daily basis, looking for the ideal combination.

I was also looking for the ideal way to use my foundation before we destroyed our reputation in the community. While we couldn't match the first gala, we tried—and spent a lot of money doing it. People in Portland knew about us because of the gala, but they weren't sure exactly what all of it was going toward. Truth is, we didn't, either. The last thing I wanted my donors to think is that they were just funding a gala.

All of that upset people in the area running other Parkinson's programs. They weren't unhappy we joined the fight, they just wanted to see what we were going to do next now that we'd drawn so much attention—and when it became clear we didn't have a concise plan they saw it as more of a negative than a positive. That hurt.

They weren't the only ones coming for us. By the third gala, we found ourselves $300,000 in debt, coincidentally almost the same amount we had been able to donate to Michael's foundation after the first one. At that point, I had a choice: pay off the $300,000 out of my pocket and shutter the foundation, or pay off the $300,000 out of my pocket and find a more cost-effective way to help the Parkinson's community.

Both on a personal and a program level, I went back to my roots—getting physical. I hired a new director for the foundation and continued to hold an annual gala, but dropped the golf tournament and scaled back in other ways. I knew from my first couple of years with the disease how much misinformation there was out there about Parkinson's and how to treat it, so we channeled our energy into creating a website that provided sensible and medically supported ways for anyone with PD to improve their quality of life and connect with the PD community. I knew firsthand how tempting it was to isolate out of embarrassment or fear and how destructive that could be, too.

Telling the world I had PD put me in touch with a lot of other people who have it and what I found pretty quickly is that a lot of us are still pretty active, but the exercise programs offered were for people in wheelchairs or using walkers. Okay, so maybe we can't win this fight—but I wanted to find a way to last as many rounds as I could and I found other people who did, too.

Parkinson's comes in many forms and each person is different. There are people who have heavy tremors, like me. There are also people who have more slowness and rigidity. I have a friend who is going through that as I write this. This tells you how far I've come: I feel blessed to have the type that I have. I'm well over 15 years living with it and still can do almost everything I want to do.

As a basketball player, if I paid attention to my diet and worked out on a daily basis, I was rewarded with improvement; I was stronger, faster, and jumped higher. Parkinson's doesn't play by those rules. Even if I stayed active and ate healthy, it was still going to take some of my strength and flexibility and balance; it would just take less of it than if I sat on the couch.

I also had to accept working out in a different way, with a different purpose. Lifting weights to have a chiseled chest and bulging shoulders and rock-hard abs and thighs was out; I had to concentrate on counteracting the effects of PD. My old post-playing routine consisted of 30 or 40 minutes of cardio, leg and bicep curls, crunches for my abs, and the bench press for a strong chest. All that was taking me in the wrong direction. Parkinson's wants to close down the body, which means expansion exercises are critical. It doesn't mean you're relegated to having a flabby chest, it just means that for every chest-building exercise, you have to do three back-strengthening exercises to keep your upper body open and limber. Curls are not advisable. Lat pulldowns and mountain climbers and standing flys are all good.

The first exercise programs I found for Parkinson's patients were depressing—they focused on teaching how to get in and out of a chair or walking in a straight line. For anyone still relatively young and in the early stages of PD, they were useless. I wanted a training program that resembled a real workout, that would inspire someone with PD because it made them feel normal. So we called our program a "boot camp" and made it challenging enough that you'd work up a pretty good sweat whether you had PD or not. We formed a board of advisors to identify traditional exercises especially beneficial for someone with Parkinson's. Balance becomes an issue for anyone who has the disease—because it attacks your flexibility—so we included ladder drills and shuffles and side-to-side slides, non-contact boxing, yoga, and tai chi.

I knew better than anyone that keeping a healthy mind was as important as a healthy body. There's no getting around that the effects of Parkinson's are very visible and the natural response is to isolate or avoid letting anyone see that you're different—especially those close to you. So we created Wellness Retreats, where people with PD and their caregivers could get together and share their experiences. Why include the caregivers? We found it was important for them to connect with other caregivers so they didn't feel alone in their struggle to deal with a loved one who has PD.

We talk about some pretty intimate stuff at the retreats, including sex and bowel movements. PD medications have varying effects on both. Some drugs will put the libido to sleep and others will send it into overdrive. Someone with PD and their partner have to be ready for either one. And it's not like I'm ever going to sneak up on a girl again with these shaking limbs. I don't care how many meds you take, your shit is gonna be going wild at the thought of being intimate. It's something anyone with PD has to come to terms with, but it helps when you know you're not alone and hear how other people are doing it.

Michael J. Fox does a good job of making Parkinson's look less demoralizing than it is. He's really funny and charming, but make no mistake: it's not a cheery disease. It sucks. I've seen the times when it even had him down. It's okay if you make it okay, but that takes work. Sometimes even that isn't enough. I saw couples who looked truly happy and a year later he or she was gone. They couldn't hack it. I can't blame them. What I heard a lot was, "I didn't sign up for this." My thought has always been: *None of us did.* But anyone with Parkinson's will admit one of their greatest fears is their partner jumping ship. Since my second divorce, it's been hard to develop another relationship out of fear I'll fall in love and then become such a burden that the person leaves.

The gala and the boot camps introduced me to Parkinson's patients like me—relatively young, still active, searching for a way to maintain a normal life as long as possible. Sharing our struggles with that helped, so we formed a local group called "The Shakers" and met about once a month. One of the things we talked about a lot is having people treat us like invalids. We all still had enough pride that it felt like an insult when someone offered to do something for us that we could easily do for ourselves. One day I got the wild idea that we should do something really bold to prove to ourselves and everyone around us that just because we had Parkinson's didn't mean we were disabled. After hearing some non-Parkinson's buddies talk about their adventures climbing a couple of local mountains, Mt. Hood and Mt. Rainier, I proposed to the Shakers group that we climb Mt. St. Helens. It's challenging enough that you need to get a permit, but not so challenging that it requires technical equipment. It's more than eight miles up and back and nearly 5,000 feet in elevation.

Charisse, my foundation director at the time, got in touch with Vincent "Enzo" Simone, a former musician and politician who one day decided to change his life and start climbing mountains to raise funds for research into diseases after his mother and father-in-law were diagnosed with Alzheimer's and Parkinson's within three months of each other. His biggest project, *Ten Mountains Ten Years*, became an award-winning movie narrated by Anne Hathaway, with Bruce Springsteen providing the soundtrack. I happened to catch a screening of it and was blown away by how inspiring it was.

When I told Simone what I wanted to do, he was happy not only to organize it but to assemble a film crew to document it, thinking that our climb could be inspirational to people with PD around the world.

Those first nine months of retirement had done a lot of damage to me physically. I was nowhere near ready for a 12-hour climb. The anticipation of facing Mount St. Helens stirred that same feeling in me as getting ready for Pat Riley's "Tens." Portland has some pretty hilly terrain, so Allison—she did the climb with me—and I trained by walking up and down the hills in our neighborhood. By the day of the climb, I had my weight down to 280 pounds, after letting it balloon to well over 300.

The Shakers—me, Brian Ruess, Hadley Ferguson, Kelly Sweeney, Mike Decker, and Barney Hyde—along with Enzo and our significant others, gathered on a late-summer day at 4:30 AM at the base and started up the mountain, our headlamps bobbing in the dark. The first four miles consist of a trail through a shady wooded area, followed by four miles of a barren rocky trail snaking through boulders, followed by a quarter-mile of ash. All of it going up.

When I proposed the climb, I overlooked the fact that guys my size are generally not built to be mountain climbers. About halfway to the top, I had sweated completely through my jacket. The higher we went, though, the colder it got and I found myself shivering uncontrollably. Enzo offered me his jacket and I didn't hesitate, stripping mine off and throwing his on, even though it was far too small and split up the back when I put it on. He saved me. I would've had no choice but to turn around or suffer hypothermia long before I reached the top.

There's a point among the boulders where I could see the summit, or at least the line where the mountain meets the sky, and it gave me a burst of faith that I was going to make it. After another 30 minutes of climbing, though, I looked up and it didn't feel as if I had moved any closer and that excitement turned into a sour feeling in my gut. Watching the video crew guys hop from rock to rock while lugging their equipment worked as motivation, though—damned if I was going to come up short when these cats were jumping around carrying all that equipment.

That last quarter-mile might've been the worst, because now the top looked so close I felt as if I could almost reach out and touch it. But every step I took, I slid back at least half a step in the ash. I was the last one to reach the top and normally my competitive spirit would've bristled at that, but it gave me the chance to see everyone sitting together, enjoying the spectacular view and the bond of accomplishment I had known so many times on an NBA court. To feel it on that mountaintop with a group of PD warriors and the people closest to them was an experience I'll never forget.

It will also go down as, physically, the hardest thing I've ever done. Pat's Miami Heat practices were brutal, but I knew we were going to be there no more than four hours. I didn't know how long I'd be on that damn mountain.

What I also quickly discovered is that going down is far more challenging than going up. The idea of standing on the summit is inspiring in a way that getting back to the parking lot is not. For anyone with balance issues, going downhill can also be trickier than going up. Friends of mine told me to bring a bag so I could ride down the sections of glacier in the higher regions on my butt, but after seeing three- and four-foot gaps in the ice that dropped into nothingness, there was no chance I was doing that. So walk back down it was.

At one point, my friend Brian was struggling so badly on the way down he thought he might need to be airlifted off the mountain. Enzo talked him through it. I had a moment like that as well after we dropped below the tree line. "If the cars aren't around this next bend," I said, "you're going to have to get a four-wheeler and cart me the rest of the way."

The cars weren't around the next bend, but I kept going. When I finally did see the car, I almost started crying. I was so tired, I climbed into the back of the Escalade, laid down in the back with my feet hanging out of the window and didn't move all the way home. I wasn't alone. I don't remember who it was, but someone in the Shakers group joked, "Next time, Brian, let's go whitewater rafting—because I'd rather drown than have to come back down another mountain."

I ended up having the toenails on both of my big toes removed and it took a couple of days to recover, but in the big picture, those seemed like small payments for what we accomplished. As we worked on editing the film and creating a documentary about the climb, the value of what we did started to dawn on me. It meant a lot personally for everyone who did it, because it raised our sense of normalcy, but I also began to think of what it would mean for someone with Parkinson's in Dallas or Miami to see us doing that climb. Living in Portland, we take hiking and mountain climbing as something that everybody does, so the feat didn't seem all that special. Seeing and hearing people comment about it, though, made me realize the statement it made about the way most people think of anyone with Parkinson's and their limitations. Mountains come in all kinds of different forms and this was a message to anyone who had PD: Find your mountain and climb it.

My one regret in making the video is that my ego got in the way. I let them use only a couple of shots of me looking weak or struggling to keep my balance, and only one shot where I had this stone-faced look. I now realize for people with Parkinson's watching it, seeing me struggle and still make it to the top—and back down—is what they could relate to and what they needed to see.

I'm not a do-what-I-say-not-what-I-do guy. I believe in walking the walk, not just talking the talk. But I also have to be honest—while I promote and support the benefits of exercise and good nutrition on Parkinson's, I have struggled keeping my own advice. Not having the pleasure of dunking a basketball, among other things, has increased my appetite for the things I can do that *do* make me feel good—pie, ice cream, and other shakes being at the top of the list. After we transitioned from holding local boot camps to training instructors to teach them in various locations across the country, issues with my feet flared up. That, combined with an unusually long stretch of cold, rainy Portland weather, took me out of my exercise routine. A look in a full-length mirror one day convinced me I needed to reconnect with Dodd or the next time I spoke about exercise and nutrition I'd have a room full of people rolling their eyes at me.

I mentioned earlier that if you are loyal to Pat Riley he will be forever loyal to you. That has continued to be true. In 2017, the Heat held a Shake It 'Til You Make It event and honored me with another video describing what I meant to the organization and my battle with Parkinson's. The team also donated another $25,000 to my foundation.

While I was there, Pat put his arm around my waist and noticed that I was carrying quite a bit of extra weight. "You know what you need to do?" Riley asked.

My heart was still conditioned to beat a little faster any time Riley made a request. "What?" I asked.

"I want you to come back down to Miami. Let Bill [Foran] have you for a month. He can get you back. You've done let yourself go a bit." He knew that carrying too much weight wasn't good for my knees, my mental state, or my fight against PD. I wanted to get back in shape, but I wasn't sure I was up for what Bill would put me through—so I gave myself an out.

"You're right, Coach," I said. "But I think I'm going to get back together with Dodd."

Riley nodded. He knew Dodd. His wife, Chris, had hired Dodd at one point and came back "absolutely ripped," Riley said, smiling.

"Dodd can do it, too."

Here's the crazy part—Riley and I were talking on a balcony. I looked over the edge and who is there, looking up at me through these dark shades like some buff undercover cop? Dodd.

I had not seen him in almost seven years. In my head, I hadn't fully committed to working out with him again; that's not something you do casually. There was no avoiding it now. He was waiting for me. "What's up, Dodd?" I asked as we exchanged a bro hug.

"I knew you were going to come to Miami at some point," he said. "Brother, God told me it's time to get it right."

That, of course, meant getting me right. I couldn't argue. My weight had crept up to nearly 350 pounds. After seeing Dodd, I went back to Portland and made plans to go down to Miami for a year to work out with him.

The stay ended up being only six months. Dodd was working intensely with Jennifer Lopez, which meant having to fly up to New York and other places to accommodate her schedule. Between that, his other celebrity clients, and his uncertainty about how much he could push me because of the Parkinson's, it gave us an excuse not to go as hard as we had before. We did enough to get me moving again and I dropped more than 30 pounds, making the trip worth it, but it wasn't the same. The good that came out of it, other than reconnecting with Dodd, is I realized I needed to find a way to stay motivated on my own, that boot camps and sessions with a personal trainer, however long, were temporary solutions. I needed to develop a daily routine I could sustain.

Exercise was not the only thing on my to-do list that I had been putting off. There was also sitting down with all of my kids and coming clean on exactly how they all came to become mine. My relationship with their moms wasn't always great and I understood why—a man who has a child with a woman but chooses to be married to someone else is going to create hard feelings. I did that twice. But I never had any intention of doubling down on the pain or hurt I caused by not being part of any of my kids' lives, no matter what it took or how mad their moms might be at me for choosing Gina.

And, trust me, they were plenty mad at times. I spent countless hours and a ton of money in attorney fees assuring I could spend time with my kids as they were growing up. After Allison and I divorced, she moved back to Illinois with our two sons, Max and Brian. I made a point of flying out regularly to spend time with them or having all three come out to see me. I made sure Jonavan and Amani knew that I would fly them to Portland to hang with their brothers and sisters whenever they wanted, which they did a lot.

It was important, too, though, that I was on good terms with the moms. As challenging as it may have been at times, I genuinely like being friends with them now. Amanda, Monica, Gina, and Allison are all great moms and our kids are a reflection of that.

After we moved back to Portland, Gina traveling the world on her Zumba tours had given me plenty of time by myself to connect with our four kids. I got to do that again during the COVID-19 pandemic, with everyone except the "littles," as I like to call Brian and Max and Jonavan, who couldn't leave Canada. Sitting back, listening to their conversations, and watching them have fun together actually made me grateful for the pandemic. It was one such moment that convinced me I needed to clear the air with them about how they came to be brothers and sisters.

My daughter, Maliah, had a steady boyfriend at the time. Her sister casually asked what she thought about another boy and Maliah shrugged and said, "I guess he's cute." That's when I decided to tease her.

"Maliah, I didn't take you for the kind who would have a boyfriend and talk about another boy," I said.

Maliah couldn't believe I'd talk to her about fidelity. She looked at me in disbelief. "What? What about—" and she pointed to Jonavan.

Touché.

She didn't mean it to hurt Jonavan's feelings; it was a shot at me. But it left me wondering exactly how the four older boys felt about me and their relationship with each other. I sat the four of them down in my living room one summer day and, one by one, came clean.

"Amani, your mom and I were really young," I said. "She gave me a ride home, we had a few beers, one thing led to another, and that's how you came along. Me and your mom used to fight like cats and dogs over you, but it's only because we both love you."

"I remember," he said.

"Jonavan, me and your mom had a relationship when we shouldn't have. We met before I was married but we kept the relationship going even after that, and that's how you came to be."

"Jaydon and Elijah, your mom is the love of my life, but she went through a lot of shit with me. I'm always going to have a place in my heart for her because she gave me you two and your sisters."

"Anything else any of you want to know?"

They looked at each other, shrugged, and went back to what they had been doing.

That none of them said anything didn't surprise me. If there was anything they wanted to know, I figured they wouldn't want to bring it up in front of each other because they wouldn't want to run the risk of offending one of their brothers. The truth is, they don't seem to be the least bit self-conscious about any of it. It was extremely embarrassing for me at the time to have two women pregnant—not once, but twice—but the benefit was that Amani and Elijah, and then Jaydon and Jonavan, were able to grow up as particularly close brothers.

What I'm most impressed by is my boys are not like me— they've learned from my mistakes. Their attitude about messing around is essentially this: *Your dad did it, you did it, no way I'm going to do it.* That's not something I tried to force-feed them;

I didn't feel I had the right to ask them to live by principles I didn't at their age. Luckily, they got it all on their own.

Amani and Jaydon organized a peaceful protest in Portland and arranged for Michael Fesser, a 48-year-old local Black man targeted and falsely arrested by local police, to meet with the police chief and discuss reform. They both spoke eloquently about their experiences of racism in our town, West Linn—experiences I didn't have, I am sure, because I was a Blazer. I couldn't help but think about my sons fearlessly seeking a reality in their hometown much different than I knew in mine.

I'm also grateful that they've all chosen to stay close to me and close to each other. Gina deserves a lot of credit for that second part. When Amani and Jonavan were with us, she treated them as she did all of our kids and when they couldn't be with us she encouraged me to go see them. She could've been resentful toward their mothers because of my relationship with them, but instead she supported everyone trying to get along for the sake of the kids.

Elijah lives with me as I write this, as does Jaydon when he's not up at Oregon State in Corvallis, going to school and playing football. Amani has a house in Portland. Jonavan has been living up in Vancouver but has plans to move to Portland as soon as we can get him dual citizenship; the novel coronavirus put the brakes on getting that done. I share Maliah and Anaya with Gina and they're with me every other week.

After everything, I wake up most days feeling blessed. There are times I'll lapse into thinking, *Why me?* Those are the times when I let phone calls go to voicemail and don't answer the door. But instead of days, my bouts of isolation only last hours. My kids being around me makes it hard to stay that way for long. They keep me both honest and grateful.

I've also confided in enough people about my many shortcomings that they call me on them now. (Raphael, who also lives in Portland now, is one of them.) More important, I appreciate it and listen when they do.

While I feel lucky that I've been able to maintain a pretty high quality of life, the disease has noticeably progressed, and it's left its mark. I had to have one of my toes partially amputated to get rid of an infection that wouldn't go away and threatened to take my whole foot. Treating the infection forced me to miss the retirement ceremony for Miami Heat legend Dwyane Wade, because my doctor advised me not to travel. I have bouts of lockjaw, or temporomandibular disorder (TMJ). I sometimes go for days when I can't sleep. My memory, both long and short term, has gaps, by-products of both PD and the medication to control it.

When I focus on what PD has taken away from me, it drags me down a dangerous rabbit hole. I start thinking about what it's going to take next. My ability to drive a car? To walk without assistance? To dress myself? To swallow?

That's when I have to remind myself that I saw Parkinson's as a death sentence when I was first diagnosed and that, almost 15 years later, I'm still here—and so many people who have been part of my journey since my diagnosis, who I thought were so blessed not to have what I have, are no longer here.

Dr. Newman, it turns out, had hip cancer when I met him and finally succumbed to it in 2016. He was 58. Philippe, after being diagnosed with cancer, moved back to France in 2011 and had himself placed in an induced coma; I spoke to him 36 hours before he died and we were able to say our goodbyes. He was 44.

My Lakers' teammate who seemed invincible, Kobe Bryant, died in a helicopter crash with his daughter, Gianna, in January 2020. He was 41 and she was 13. My dad, Tommy Grant, lost his battle with cancer in the spring of 2020. Enzo died in May of 2020. He was 53.

Losing every one of them made me wonder how much time I had left, but the death of Jerome Kersey might've hit me hardest because we had grown especially close the last few years and it was so unexpected. A blood clot he didn't even know he had in his left calf broke loose and travelled all the way up to his lungs, causing a pulmonary thromboembolism. He was 52. I was in downtown Portland at a jazz festival when my phone started blowing up with calls and text messages. My son Jaydon heard about Jerome's death before I did and called me crying.

I reached out to another former Blazer, Terry Porter, who had already heard, too, and was taking it just as hard.

I couldn't help but think about Romeo being the first former teammate I confided in about my tremor and how he treated it as no big deal; we had made plans the day before he died to get together to play golf.

How do I reconcile that they're gone and I'm still here? It was their time. My time is going to come, too. There's a way to acknowledge that without sinking into a depression over it. It's actually useful, because it makes me recognize that I, like everyone else, have an expiration date. I used to think, *I'll live until I'm 80 or so, they'll come out with some anti-aging formulas and maybe I'll add another 40 years, get to 120.* And I used to live that way. Every day is different now. How my meds react with my morning cup of coffee, the mood created by my ever-fluctuating brain chemistry, the stiffness brought on by Parkinson's along with the aging scar tissue in all my surgically repaired joints can go a long way to charting what kind of day it will be before I've even rubbed the sleep out of my eyes. But then I shuffle down the stairs, sit at the kitchen table listening to the happy chatter of my gang of teenagers, and it never fails to put a smile on my face. I made some dumb decisions, shattered a few hearts, and fought a few extra battles because of them, and yet wound up with this good-hearted crew that is happy to call me their dad.

On top of that, I have a purpose. Being a spokesman for Parkinson's is a challenge for me in that I am more than willing to use my profile and connections to help the cause, but I'm uncomfortable accepting any credit or thinking of myself as a great person for doing it. There's a fine line between being visible and drawing attention to myself. I was fierce as a player and played with my heart on my sleeve and fury in my eyes, but I was never a showboat; I don't want to be a PDPD—Parkinson's Disease Prima Donna.

When I've really got it all together, though, I take PD as God's way of saying he believed I was strong enough not only to deal with it, but to help others deal with it, too. When I'm thinking that way, I take every setback or challenge given to me by PD as a lesson meant to be shared with someone else that might add a few extra quality days to their clock.

I wish I could tell you I think like that all of the time; I don't. My initial reaction to someone in my life dying is to feel bad for them and their loved ones and think, *I have the same thing coming! I don't want to die!*

I've had that thought enough times now that I know how to move past it. I've come to understand that when I start worrying about dying, it means there must be something going on in my life that I need to take care of and am avoiding.

I realize that everyone thinks about their mortality as they get older. My friends who don't have PD assure me that they, too, have thoughts about what old age will take from them and how much longer they have to live. The only difference for me is I started thinking about all that one day out of the blue, at 36 years old, sitting in Dr. Nutt's office—and every single day since.

When I'm in that good place, though, I actually appreciate PD for making me aware of that ticking clock, because it pushes me to go do the things I love—fish, exercise, hang with my friends and family—and appreciate that I get to do them today, without worrying if I will be able to do them tomorrow.

I was fortunate enough to be asked to speak at the 2016 World Parkinson Congress. It was there that a mother approached me and said her 14-year-old daughter wanted "to meet the Blazer who had Parkinson's." It stopped me in my tracks—for the first time, I heard the disease sound like a badge of honor.

Being perfectly comfortable up on stage in an enormous room speaking to a large audience made me realize something else about Parkinson's: I had been so focused on what it was taking away from me, I missed what it has given. Once terrified of being drafted because it would mean going up on a stage to shake hands and say a few words to a room full of strangers, I now looked forward to speaking to audiences all over the country and telling my story.

Without Parkinson's I never would've climbed Mt. St. Helens. I never would've seen that view. I never would've learned I was capable of that. I didn't join a team, I helped create one.

And I didn't do it for money or fame or recognition, but as an act of faith, of service and love for anyone with their own mountain to climb.

Having Parkinson's also has changed my view of relationships. I don't know if I'll ever get married again, but if I do it's going to be in a church, with bridesmaids and groomsmen, and we're going to get all dressed up.

It took writing this book to discover that I had it twisted. Here I thought I had it all and my disease was slowly but surely robbing me.

The truth?

Basketball gave me a life; Parkinson's taught me how to live it.